D1711162

The
Naturopathic
Approach to
Fertility

Dr. Julissa Hernandez, ND, CNHP

Ingram   12/17   2/7/18

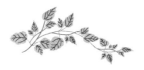

Dedication

This long-awaited book, a dream realized, is dedicated first and foremost to, God, my Creator, and to my one and only beautiful Son. I am honored he chose me to be his mother.

To my loving family, and friends, who have always given me so much love and infinite support, forever believing in my dreams and my work. To all of my adoring patients through the years, who have kept me feeling blessed each and every day with their healing and overwhelmed with joy to be doing what I love.

And to all of you, my dear readers, for allowing me the opportunity to be a part of fulfilling your dream of having a healthy baby and for helping you achieve overall healing and optimum health.

This is a divine gift you give to me.

~ Thank You ~

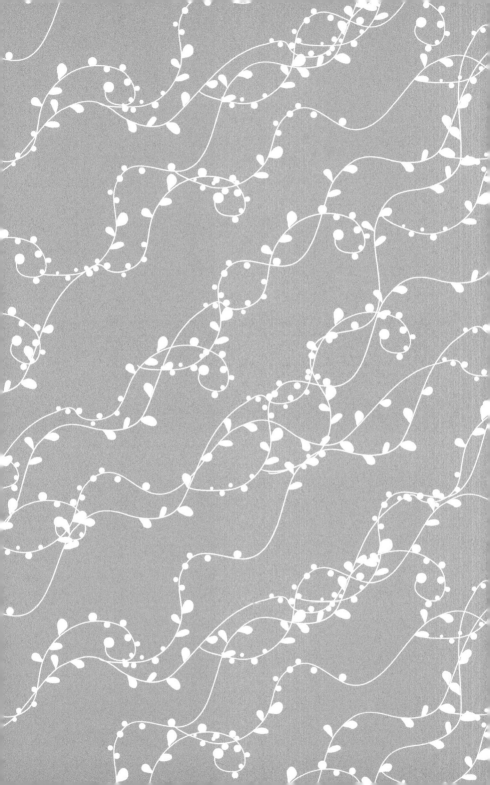

Table of Contents

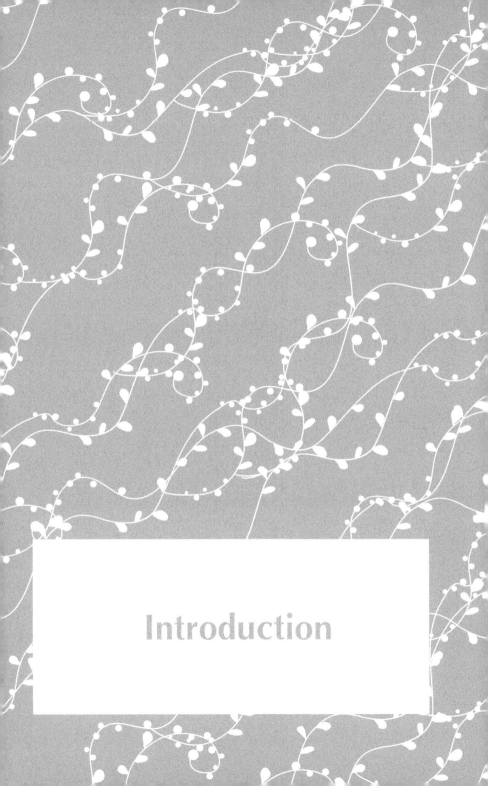

Introduction

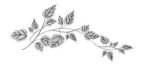

Becoming a parent is one of the most exhilarating joys and one of the happiest moments of life! To touch, hold, and breathe in the delicate scent of a little baby of your own creation... no words can truly capture the rapture one feels in every cell of ones body when that day arrives! You know that from that very moment, your life will most definitely never be the same. Having a child will bring you the blessings of infinite love.

This is what I wish for you and your partner. In The Naturopathic Approach to Fertility, I share the same steps I have recommended time and again over my 21 years in practice as a naturopathic doctor for couples yearning to become parents. Why am I so confident in this process? Because although I may not be able to speak for every naturopathic doctor, every couple who has come to me with fertility challenges has achieved a healthy pregnancy after following my recommendations and suggested individual programs. That is a 100 percent success rate! Allow me to help you achieve this dream.

If you are reading this book, you have most likely encountered challenges getting pregnant. Sadly, more and more couples today are having problems conceiving a child naturally. Fertility challenges affect both sexes, ranging from a number of reasons for women aside from their age to the fact that men have shown a more than a 50 percent decrease in sperm count over the last 60 to 75 years. Many couples invest in infertility treatments, such as chemical drugs and invasive procedures, that leave them childless and emotionally and financially drained. However, many couples haven't considered a holistic approach to fertility.

This may sound like a New Age idea. And yet, it means there is a widespread need for women and men struggling with fertility to open up their horizons and take naturopathic methods seriously. In The Naturopathic Approach to Fertility, couples seeking to become parents through natural conception will gain a comprehensive understanding of this alternative to western medicine. What's more, you will learn about how certain herbs and roots can help you overcome some of the issues preventing you from making a baby.

My heartfelt desire is to help you become a parent. One of my greatest joys is to know that I have helped a loving couple conceive the baby they so wished for. In this book, I share stories of couples, patients of mine, who tried numerous times to make a baby and failed—until we all found each other. In their stories, you may see reflections of your own difficulties and struggles with conception.

Let me take you through a brief journey of what this book will deliver, how it will enlighten you and give you comfort and hope:

Why should you consider a naturopathic approach to fertility?

In chapter one, you'll learn the differences between conventional, allopathic medicine and the holistic view of naturopathic medicine. Conventional fertility methods are distressing, exhausting, and extremely expensive. Plus, there are many unfortunate side effects, from the likelihood of multiple births to an increased risk in birth defects and abnormalities. To aggravate matters, sex for conception through conventional methods can become regimented and mechanical. By embracing the naturopathic alternative to conception, you will learn how to avoid the emotional, physical, and financial burdens associated with conventional tactics and technologies. You'll make the precious child you so wish for without increased risk of abnormalities. And you will do it without sacrificing intimacy. Instead, you will grow closer to each other, embracing each other's love more deeply, and using this as a catalyst to make your very own tiny creation.

From anemia, to hormonal imbalances, to lifestyle habits, the list of obstacles to fertility is long and often surprising. Chapter two details the most common causes of fertility challenges, offering a comprehensive, eye-opening overview. Of course, my dear readers, my goal is to provide you with the natural alternative solutions to overcoming each and every one of the fertility challenges detailed. You will find herbal solutions scattered throughout the book. Most importantly, this is the chapter in which I share the Essential Female Herbal Fertility Program and the Essential Male Herbal Fertility Program, which you and your partner need to follow until you achieve your successful pregnancy.

Would you believe that ibuprofen—which I am sure many of you have used on occasion, if not take regularly—can be a contributing factor to your fertility problems?

Yes. Believe it. Chapter three discusses the all-too-common practice of using pharmaceutical medications and how these drugs can hinder your ability to conceive a child. In this chapter, you'll find facts on the hazards of common pain relievers and more shocking information about the drugs, both prescription and over-the-counter, you must stop using to increase your fertility.

Anger, fear, unresolved forgiveness, and unconscious thoughts... Did you know that holding onto such emotional baggage could be hindering the body from responding positively to conceiving a child?

In chapter four, you will move beyond physical matters to focus on your thoughts and feelings. As you'll come to understand, harboring specific negative emotions for a prolonged period of time, and even negative thinking in general, can take a toll on your fertility. With the information and tools I offer in this chapter, you will be able to overcome inner turmoil and let go of whatever burdens you or your partner have been carrying. You must both find inner peace to be sure your bodies are open to receive the baby you see in your future.

Chapter five delves into the crucial role hormones play in fertility—for men as well as women. You'll learn about common issues of estrogen dominance and low progesterone in women and low testosterone and other hormonal challenges in men. You'll also learn how to restore hormonal balance and fertility with my natural herbal therapy recommendations.

Did you ever think poor circulatory system health could affect your fertility?

If proper blood flow is not reaching your reproductive system, then it could be lacking essential nutrients and oxygen that could be contributing to its weakened state. Chapter six will shed light on what symptoms you and your partner could be experiencing—think varicose veins, poor erections, and more—that indicate your circulatory system needs additional support. You'll also find additional herbal therapy solutions to overcome these challenges and in turn increase your fertility chances.

Did you ever have a sexually transmitted disease (STD)? Are you still suffering from an STD today? Is your partner?

As you'll learn in chapter seven, some STDs can cause scarring or trauma of the reproductive system, which also plays a factor into the health of the woman—or the man—making a baby. If this could be you, then be relieved to know I touch upon this issue in great depth and offer herbal solutions.

Men, your role in making a baby is just as important as a woman's. Your state of health is crucial to your love's ability to conceive and have a healthy pregnancy, and so I have devoted a chapter to you. In chapter eight, you'll learn important facts about men's reproductive health—from understanding sperm count to sperm quality, mobility, motility, and normal sperm formation. I'll discuss what needs to be done to double your sperm count naturally, along with other steps to make you as fertile as possible.

Are you and your partner coffee lovers?

That caffeine habit can be detrimental to your fertility. Chapter nine focuses on how your everyday lifestyle practices affect your chances of conception. Even little things—such as drinking just a cup of the wrong brew to get you 'functioning' in the morning, exposure to second-hand smoke, and not getting enough sleep—can play a huge role in making a baby. Be open to making some changes so that you can finally conceive and, at the same time, so you can both pass on healthy genes to your child.

What about the foods you eat on a daily basis? Do you feel you have a healthy diet? Or do you know you should eat healthier?

In chapter ten, I discuss how healthy prenatal nutrition should start long before the moment of conception. You'll learn what to eat and what not to eat (fact: some foods double the likelihood of delayed conception) to bolster fertility.

There are many charts and apps out there to help a woman determine when she is at her peak fertility and most likely to get pregnant. It can all be very confusing. So, how does a woman gauge her own most fertile time of the month naturally?

In chapter eleven, I share the simple, dependable method I teach couples in my practice. Every woman will learn how to accurately calculate ovulation from the first day of her period—no matter how long her menstrual cycle is. And couples will learn precisely when, what sexual positions to use, and how often in order to enjoy sex to achieve conception. Yes, lovemaking for baby-making should be pleasurable!

Lastly, you'll find a glossary with detailed information on the herbs I recommend throughout the book. It is a spotlight on herbs and roots proven to help female and male bodies heal reproductive health problems.

So be prepared, my dear friends. This is a journey we will take together, that you two—and I—will cherish when the outcome is holding a precious baby. It will be an honor to help you both achieve this, and I feel blessed to have this opportunity to be a part of such a life-changing miracle in your lives. Thank you. And now, let us begin...

Dr. Julissa

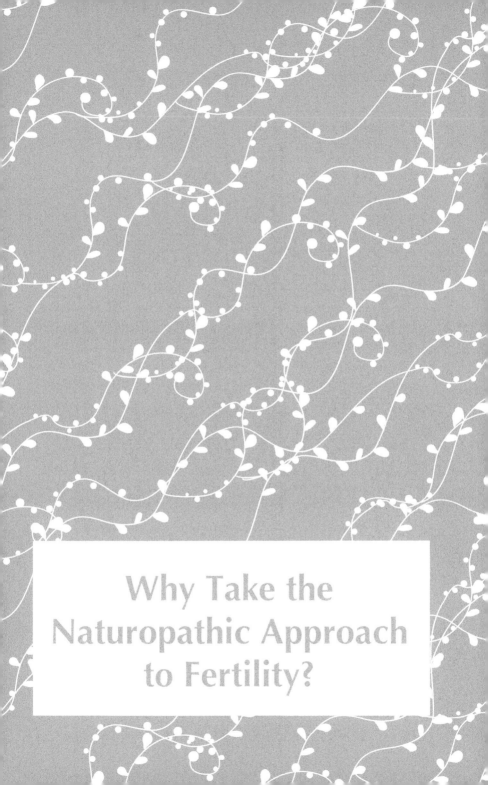

Why Take the
Naturopathic Approach
to Fertility?

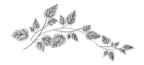

Since the birth of the world's first "test-tube baby" in 1978, there have been astounding medical and technical advances in treating fertility challenges. Today, a woman with a fertility problem, working with an allopathic, conventional medical doctor can get a prescription for a drug like Clomid, which works by stimulating an increase in the hormones that support ovulation.

If that fails, she might choose to invest in assisted reproductive technology (ART) interventions like in vitro fertilization (IVF), or even be put on a waiting list for a whole uterine transplant. For a man with a fertility problem, conventional medical solutions include testosterone-boosting drugs and surgical interventions. With all these cutting-edge options, why would a couple yearning and struggling to make a baby together choose the naturopathic path to conception?

Over my 21 years in practice as a Doctor of Naturopathy (ND), I have been thrilled—truly, exhilarated—to help numerous couples overcome their fertility problems. Again and again, couples have come to me after trying conventional fertility methods, after suffering side effects from prescription drugs, and after wasting tens of thousands of dollars on IVF. Again and again, frustrated, desperate couples have realized their cherished dream of becoming biological parents, of creating their own tiny, precious miracle, by embracing naturopathic approaches. One such young lady named Karen, 33 years of age at the time and married, came to see me for a fertility consultation, alone, on May 11, 2011. She had undergone two expensive IVF procedures, which both culminated in unsuccessful pregnancies.

The first procedure, as she explained, weakened her uterine walls causing a miscarriage. Upon the second IVF procedure, she miscarried again. She described not only the emotional pain of undergoing two heartbreaking failed procedures but also the physical pain leading up to them. Prior to each IVF, she had to constantly inject herself with subcutaneous medications, those injected into the fat deposits just under the skin, and intramuscular medications, those injected directly into the muscle—an excruciating ordeal.

After the second failure, shedding countless tears of sadness, Karen and her husband had a discussion and decided to take the naturopathic approach. Her husband was adamant about not allowing her to go through such discomfort and distress again.

Despite all the news about high-tech breakthroughs (you've undoubtedly heard raves about the latest rage: egg cryopreservation), conventional medical treatments for fertility problems don't always work. And even when they do, they take a terrible toll on a couple's physical, emotional, and financial health. To put it bluntly, allopathic approaches to fertility are traumatic.

According to various medical experts, the most common side effects for women taking fertility-stimulating medications include:

- *Bloating and cramping*
- *Painful breast tenderness*
- *Persistent headaches and migraines*
- *Heavy vaginal bleeding*
- *Pelvic pain*
- *Blood in the urine*
- *Hot flashes and mood swings*
- *An increased risk of fevers spiking to 100.5 degrees Fahrenheit.*

In addition, these drugs may cause ovarian hyper-stimulation syndrome (OHSS). This syndrome sets in after a woman has used injectable hormone medications during in vitro fertilization (IVF).

These medications stimulate the ovaries to produce eggs; however, it is difficult to say how much medication a woman may need. Too much medication can lead to OHSS, causing the ovaries to become swollen and painful.

Along with this severe development, some women notice rapid weight gain, abdominal pain, shortness of breath, and vomiting. Even more distressing is that OHSS can occur spontaneously.

IVF and other forms of Assisted Reproductive Technology (ART) come with their own list of serious, distressing symptoms. They include:

- *Decreased urinary frequency*
- *Nausea or vomiting*
- *Feelings of dizziness or faintness, as well as shortness of breath*
- *Dramatic, rapid weight gain — 10 pounds or more within three to five days*
- *Severe stomach pains and bloating*
- *Risks of bleeding, infection, and damage to the bladder or bowel.*

What's more, with many forms of ART—but IVF in particular—women who achieve conception face an increased likelihood of miscarriage (as exemplified in Karen's story) or multiple births with increased risk of premature delivery and low birth weight. Beyond the medical risks and complications, the process of investing money, time, and hope in conventional medical fertility treatments puts severe stresses on a couple's relationship and resources. Emotional distress and psychological problems are highly common, especially if IVF has been repeatedly unsuccessful.

Many insurance plans do not provide coverage for medical allopathic fertility treatment, and IVF is expensive. On average, nationally, a "fresh" IVF cycle costs $12,000 before medications, which typically run another $3,000 to $5,000. After all the suffering and financial strain, IVF results in a surprising low rate of live births. According to research published in *The Lancet*, less than 14 percent of women who undergo IVF treatment achieve their dream of giving birth to a live baby. The birth success rate decreases with a woman's age and with each repeated IVF cycle. To add to an expectant mother's heartache, the rate of miscarriage for pregnancy through IVF is 20 to 30 percent greater than pregnancy through natural conception.

Why take the naturopathic approach to fertility? There are so many reasons—enough to fill this book! First and foremost, the answer is because it works. I can joyously say that my success rate with my fertility patients in the past 21 years in practice has been *100 percent*. I have never had a couple come to me for help in conceiving a child, who—after continuing their designated step-by-step program, following all the recommended herbal therapies, lifestyle changes, dietary changes, and suggestions—left me childless, bitter about wasting time and money on a naturopathic approach, and heartbroken.

In today's digital age of instant access to abundant information, people are much more aware of and knowledgeable about health and medical matters. Many have realized they must take their health into their own hands instead of following an allopathic, conventional medical doctor's orders without question, acting as mindless robots, and subjecting their bodies to harsh chemicals, invasive procedures, and often unnecessary, if not severe and damaging, side effects. It is a joy to see how aware people are today about other options. Naturopathy, alternative medicine, is becoming the medicine of choice. Preventing disease is considered very important to most people today. Many find that they have exhausted themselves with second and third opinions from conventional doctors with no resolution, only to finally find a solution within the realm of alternative, natural, naturopathic medicine.

As a child, I heard talk of herbal remedies to help the body heal. I watched closely as my mother, drawing on what she had learned growing up in the Dominican Republic as well as what she learned through self-education, helped others with their health problems by recommending different herbs and roots. As a teenager, I found my first love. I fell in love with natural medicine. After my studies, I became a Certified Natural Health Professional (CNHP) and, in my twenties, began consulting from my first office in New York City—in uptown Manhattan. While consulting, as we are apt to do as CNHPs, I continued to study and received my degree as a Doctor of Naturopathy. I felt ecstatic knowing I was truly on my destined life journey.

What makes natural medicine so exciting and fulfilling? Natural medicine focuses on disease prevention and helping the body to heal itself. As I explain to my patients, disease reflects a body out of balance. And the body must be fed what it is missing to help it heal itself. The main principles that distinguish natural or alternative medicine from conventional medicine come from this idea: Healing comes from *within,* not from drugs and surgery. That applies to healing fertility challenges as much as it does to healing a sore throat. When working with natural medicine, our focus is on the person and not the disease. A primary approach in naturopathy is education. I make it a priority to make sure my patients understand the reasons why they are dealing with the health challenges they face, to make them understand the root causes that brought them to this point.

This way, I have found there is little to no reluctance towards making the necessary changes within their lives to help their bodies heal. Each individual is unique. Not everyone gets treated the same way, although they may have the same symptoms. In my practice with couples struggling to conceive, I take the time to get to know each individual personally, not just take their medical history.

I talk with couples about their background, their work, their lifestyle habits, their family, their stresses, their diet, their concerns, their fears, and their dreams. As research shows, naturopaths and alternative healers spend more time with their patients and clients than allopathic, conventional medical doctors. Naturally, patients and clients are more open to discussing their problems freely in a relaxed atmosphere; they are much more joyful, relieved, and hopeful, as well as better satisfied with the quality of care, from naturopathically trained healers than they are from the conventional medical establishment.

Naturopaths are known to fall into two groups. NDs, traditionally trained naturopaths, use the Doctor of Naturopathy degree to consult with patients or clients and as an accreditation to teach, to access research, and to write. A smaller number expand their expertise by adding training in therapeutic nutrition and psychological counseling. Some also learn about specialized practices in addition to their ND title, such as: herbal therapy (becoming Masters of Herbology), massage therapy, homeopathy, hydrotherapy, chiropractic, and behavioral, as well as Ayurvedic and Oriental medicine systems. My own specialty is iridology. Holistic Iridologists like myself see the eyes as windows into the body's state of health. Iridology examines patterns, colors, and other characteristics of the iris, since, as extensive study supports, the predisposition of people's energetic values and vitality in certain areas of the body correlate with the iris nerve wreathes. The results from the iridology exam are matched to an iris chart, which will distinguish between healthy organs and those that are overactive, inflamed, or distressed. Iridology findings demonstrate a patient's susceptibility towards certain illnesses, reflects past medical problems, and predicts later health problems.

Interest, enthusiasm, and faith in naturopathy is exploding in America. Naturopathic medicine is the most sought-after and fastest-growing of all the alternative healing approaches and found to be the greatest change Americans are making in their healthcare practices. According to industry reports, the number of naturopathic physicians in practice in the United States and Canada *doubled* between 2001 and 2006. In 2013, the federal government acknowledged the safety and effectiveness of naturopathic medicine by passing a resolution designating the week of *October 7th* as Naturopathic Medicine Week to "recognize the value of naturopathic medicine in providing safe, effective, and affordable health care." Many more people each day are becoming disillusioned with conventional health care. Naturopathy is increasingly considered a wonderful alternative and sound choice that has gained respect as a credible method and healing doctrine.

Naturopathy maintains a consistent philosophy that is founded in five therapeutic principles. Even though each of their therapeutic programs is based on individual experience and individual interest, all naturopaths incorporate the following beliefs on their approach:

1. Nature is a healing and powerful force. This is the focus on the immeasurable power of the body to heal itself. Naturopaths help, facilitate, encourage, and enhance this process by teaching their patients or clients what they must do to stimulate their divine, innate healing force. First and foremost, a naturopath must vow to do no harm.

2. The patient or client is viewed as a whole. It is crucial to understand each and every individual is unique. A naturopath must take the time to understand what makes that person 'tick,' discovering their mental, physical, social, emotional and spiritual factors.

3. The focus is on understanding and finding the root cause of the health problem. Conventional medicine is known to suppress symptoms. Naturopathy is different in that it recognizes the symptoms (such as a headache or runny nose) as the body showing it is trying to heal itself.

Naturopaths delve deep to understand the underlying causes of a disease or ailment, which can come about from imbalances in the body. Some diseases, aliments, and illnesses are due to physical, emotional, spiritual, and mental imbalances.

When a person experiences emotional and spiritual imbalances, symptoms can range from unexplainable sadness, deep internal turmoil, unease, and an overall weakened state that is unable to support the body's healing process. Naturopaths are here to help patients and clients make the necessary changes to overcome this disruption of internal harmony.

4. Other underlying root causes, such as extreme stress and a poor diet, can cause symptoms in couples trying to conceive: from inflammation and fevers to low sperm mobility and miscarriages. The naturopath's job is to guide the patient or client to find the natural solution, procedure, or technique that can alleviate the stress and help stimulate healing.

I will share my favorite professional secret: the core belief of naturopathy is to educate—to pass on the wisdom and *knowledge to another so as to empower them to take their health into their own hands. Through embracing a naturopathic approach, you will be able to overcome any and all emotional and physical challenges that are known to cause imbalances within the body, and, in turn, are hindering your determined efforts to conceive a child.*

5. Prevention of disease is the best approach. You prevent illness and disease by carrying out lifestyle habits that support optimum health.

With a naturopathic approach, we can work together to feed your body what it may be missing in order for it to be strong, healthy, well-nourished, balanced, and cleared of toxins that could be hampering fertility and make sure it is ready to receive baby. We will also work on clearing out toxic emotions, such as unresolved anger and resentment, which could be hindering fertility as well.

Let's start with a general detoxifying herbal therapy combination that helps boost fertility in women and men:

1. Senna Leaf – in capsules or tea

2. Chlorophyll – in liquid or soft gels

3. Green Tea – every morning for men

4. White Tea – every morning for women

I recommend that couples commit to this detoxifying program for two weeks.

Then, both partners should continue drinking the morning teas until achieving conception. Why choose the naturopathic path to having a baby?

More than any conventional fertility treatment, naturopathy fills couples with hope. On our journey together, you will discover the fertility-enhancing benefits of simple lifestyle and dietary changes, herbal therapies, and tapping into your body's natural ability to heal. In the process, you will feel better physically and emotionally, grow closer to your partner, and find renewed faith in experiencing the miracle of parenthood.

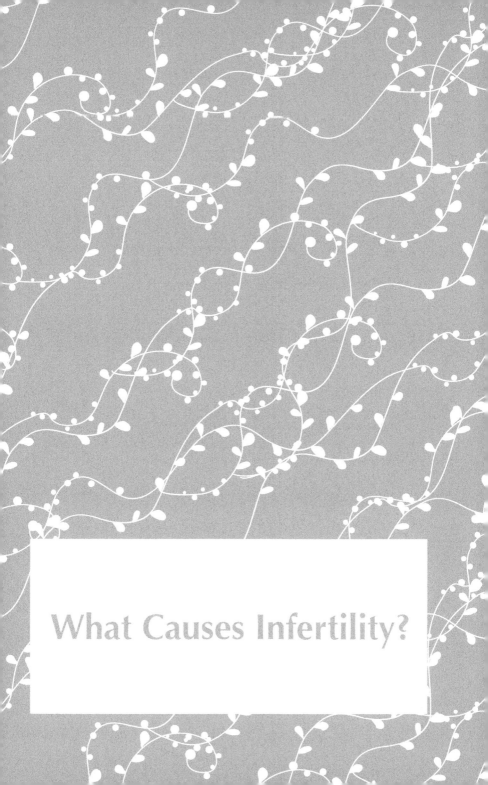

What Causes Infertility?

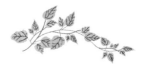

Being infertile or barren beyond hope is extremely rare. Struggling with fertility challenges, however, is extremely common. According to the latest Centers for Disease Control and Prevention (CDC) figures, of women in their prime childbearing years (between the ages of 15 and 44):

Nearly 11 percent (a staggering 6.7 million women) have impaired fecundity, or the ability to get pregnant or carry a baby to term.

Among those married, 6 percent (1.5 million women) have been pronounced infertile—that is, unable to get pregnant after at least 12 consecutive months of unprotected sex with their husband.

7.4 million women have used infertility services.

It's not just a women's issue. Among couples struggling with fertility problems, between 35 and 40 percent ultimately trace the primary cause to the woman. However, as further research shows, roughly the same number of struggling couples—between 35 and 40 percent—ultimately trace the primary cause to the man.

The list of obstacles to fertility is long and often surprising. Over my 21 years in practice as a naturopathic doctor, I have helped numerous women and men first get to the root of their fertility challenges and then work together to overcome them to fulfill their dream of bringing a precious baby into the world. To illustrate the baffling nature of fertility challenges, I'd like to share the story of one such couple, Lauren and Freddy.

Lauren had a daughter from a previous marriage. A few years after her divorce—a bitter one— she found Freddy, a wonderful man with whom she wanted to spend the rest of her life. Lauren and Freddy got married. At the time, Lauren was in her early thirties and Freddy was still in his twenties. He had no children.

While they were still in the romance phase, Lauren had an IUD inserted. Soon after they got married, Lauren and Freddy shared their desire to have a child together. Lauren's daughter, then age seven, also wanted a baby sister or brother. Lauren decided to have her IUD removed. For a few months prior to that, she had experienced general discomfort and frequent pain in the pelvic region. Her gynecologist found the culprit: Lauren's IUD had perforated her uterus. This would be a problem, her gynecologist explained, if she tried to get pregnant. So, Lauren elected to have surgery to repair her uterine wall. After recovering from her operation, Lauren was assured that she should be able to conceive without any further problems. However, she and Freddy were still having difficulty getting pregnant.

Frustrated and desperate, Lauren and Freddy came to see me in October of 2010. As I soon discovered, the cause of their fertility problem was not simply Lauren's uterine wall. Afflicted with epilepsy since childhood, Freddy had been taking the anti-seizure drug Keppra for many years. Like all drugs, Keppra is filtered through the liver. One of the body's most vital organs, the liver serves as the filter of fat, of blood, and of hormones. To boost Freddy's fertility, I had to offset the drug's side effects, strengthen his liver, and balance his hormones. Freddy was also overweight. Storing up fat is the body's way of defending against internal toxins, including prescription drugs. I began working with Freddy on detoxifying his body, improving his general fitness level, and teaching him how to eat healthier.

With Lauren, my main focus was to strengthen her uterine walls, weakened by this delicate surgery, to promote ovulation and avoid miscarriage. In addition, I began working with Lauren on an emotional level. As I helped Lauren discover, forgiving her ex-husband was absolutely vital to her overall health and her ability to conceive. As I'll discuss in more detail later in this book, unresolved emotional issues can block fertility.

After thoroughly examining and talking with both Freddy and Lauren, I recommended a fertility-enhancing program of lifestyle changes, dietary changes, and herbal therapies. They committed to following all of my recommendations. Just one month later, in November 2010, Lauren, to our joy, became pregnant. This loving couple now has a healthy, sweet little boy, and Lauren's daughter delights in the little brother she always asked her mommy for.

Lauren and Freddy's success story is uplifting and inspiring but not extraordinary. Indeed, many couples achieve their dream of bringing a baby into the world when they embrace naturopathic approaches to fertility. Unfortunately, despite growing awareness and acceptance of natural and holistic healing alternatives, large numbers of couples suffer with fertility problems and turn to traditional medicine again and again for solutions. In many cases, they do not know they have a better option.

Let's take a closer look at widespread, yet often overlooked causes of fertility problems. I'll start by focusing on underlying causes that are specific to each gender and then move on to cover fertility obstacles that couples can work on overcoming together.

Primary causes of fertility problems among women:

Gender-specific health challenges and hormonal imbalances. These range from PCOS (polycystic ovarian syndrome) and endometriosis caused by estrogen dominance to severe anemia.

Tampon use. Tampons block a woman's vaginal tract. As a result, toxic blood is not shed properly during her menstrual period and blood clots are reabsorbed into the blood and by the surrounding organs. Along with tampons, I also urge women to avoid standard commercial maxi pads. Most are laced with chlorine, which causes a vaporous effect up the vaginal tract, a damp, dark area. This causes uterine contractions, provoking cramps and heavy bleeding—to sell more pads. I recommend using only organic maxi pads.

Using an IUD (intrauterine device)—the birth control method that brought Lauren so much pain and trouble. Yes, although the facts are often refuted by research sponsored by its manufacturers, the IUD can interfere with a woman's chances of conceiving after she has it removed. Studies have linked the IUD to various fertility challenges, including vaginal inflammation. Here's one well-documented risk of having an IUD inserted: it can perforate the uterus.

Artificial vaginal lubricants. Intended to ease intercourse and increase sexual pleasure, many slick commercial creams and ointments can impede fertility. My strong advice to couples seeking to achieve conception: use ONLY natural sexual lubricants during sex—and only if truly needed. When a woman begins a naturopathic fertility program, as you'll discover firsthand, natural vaginal lubrication is enhanced.

In vitro fertilization (IVF). Evidence suggests there may be a new environmental link to failed IVF. Based on a recent study, polychlorinated biphenyls, a toxic chemical commonly known as PCB, reduces chances of live birth from IVF by 40 percent!

Relying on pain relievers—prescription or over-the-counter, all types of NSAIDs (non-steroidal anti-inflammatory drugs) and especially ibuprofen. Startling but real, this prevalent cause of fertility problems among women is widely overlooked by gynecologists as well as women themselves. I have helped many of my patients and clients recognize and overcome their unhealthy reliance on pain relievers. Many, many women routinely reach for an ibuprofen—every month for menstrual cramps, or weekly, even daily, for minor aches and pains. Here's a painful fact for women with this habit (and the men who love them) to swallow: pain relievers, particularly ibuprofen, can induce "luteinized unruptured follicle syndrome," an unfortunate syndrome in which eggs are never released for conception. In most cases, women can reclaim their fertility simply by stopping and thinking before popping NSAIDs. In chapter 3, I will talk more about medications that hinder fertility. What's more, I will offer natural treatments for aches, pains, and discomforts that target their root causes without risk of hindering your fertility.

A sperm problem—whether poor sperm formation, poor sperm quality, or low sperm count. A sperm problem is, not surprisingly, the most prevalent culprit for male fertility challenges. You'll read more about sperm matters—count, motility, mobility, and quality—in chapter 8. For now, I'll mention the connection between a healthy diet and abundant sperm. Research published in The Lancet shows that men who eat mostly organic foods produce 43 percent more sperm than those men who don't.

Gender-specific hormonal imbalances. These are not limited to low testosterone.

Estrogen dominance can also be a factor that hinders fertility in men. Heavy metal toxicity and zinc deficiency. **Zinc** is a mineral essential for sexual and reproductive system health. This vital mineral is also considered 'food' for the prostate.

The following are major causes of fertility problems that women and men have in common:

Diet. First and foremost, diet seems to be the number one factor interfering with fertility. Yes, our typical, terrible American diet: high in fast, processed foods and low in nutrition. You'll read more about the role of diet in fertility and what to eat (and not eat) to support a successful conception in chapter 10. For general health, as well as robust fertility in particular, my simple rule for everyone is: Eat More Organic Food. Your Body Is Worth It.

Caffeine. In several international studies, caffeine has been shown to hinder fertility. Here's a shocker: men and women who intake 300 milligrams or more a day of toxic caffeine, which includes many sodas as well as coffee, are

TWICE as likely to suffer from delayed conception! Coffee, even decaf, is particularly harmful to fertility. My opinion: if you and your partner drink this substance and are having trouble getting pregnant, STOP drinking coffee and soda altogether.

Stress—particularly chronic stress and anxiety. Emotional turmoil tends to cause imbalances within the body that can impede pregnancy, as study after study shows. My strong advice to every woman yearning to get pregnant: find ways to relax! Whatever feels good to you will be the best relaxation practice. Yoga, deep breathing, meditation, and taking long nature walks are all wonderfully successful relaxation techniques. Stress impedes fertility in men, too. As research affirms, stress and abnormal sperm formation and abnormal sperm production are linked. Here's a great way for stressed-out couples with fertility challenges to relax together: get side-by-side massages! Even when partners agree on their desire to make a baby, they can be divided over other issues from job pressures to financial worries. Relaxing on side-by-side massage tables, holding hands while a therapist's skilled hands work their magic to releases muscle tension, does wonders for restoring a couple's emotional connection and peace of mind.

Bacterial and viral infections—chlamydia, gonorrhea, trichomonas, candidiasis, and others. When active or flaring up, such infections can block fertility. Most often, fertility is restored once the infection is effectively treated and healed.

Smoking—whether cigarettes, cigars, or marijuana. Regularly inhaling such harmful substances can cause fertility challenges that can linger for years, even after quitting. Men who smoke may develop atherosclerosis/arteriosclerosis, a hardening of the arteries, which apart from affecting fertility can foil efforts at sustaining strong erections.

Alcohol. Like smoking, regular moderate-to-heavy drinking can hinder fertility. And, yes, men, drinking can negatively affect the virility linked to erectile function.

As you see, the causes of fertility problems are many and varied. And they're not just related to the body. Perhaps you and your partner are letting negative emotions crush your cherished dreams of pregnancy and parenthood. Over the course of trying and failing again and again, to conceive, most couples grapple with frustration, desperation, sadness, apathy, and a constant yearning to have a child together. These very feelings can contribute to fertility challenges.

I will help you to learn how to recognize and overcome your own combination of frustrating hurdles to fertility. In each chapter, you will find effective natural solutions, healing insights, easy-to-make dietary and lifestyle changes, and herbal therapy programs. Remember: the body knows how to heal itself; we just need to feed it what it is missing. You will also find comfort, joy, and hope in the many success stories I'll share—stories of couples, like Lauren and Freddy, who prove that conceiving a child is possible, despite how long you have been trying, despite the negative news you may have been given by others. And I'm certain you'll see women and men with fertility struggles similar to your own.

Regardless of your individual fertility challenges, you must begin to overcome them with a basic fertility herbal therapy program. Taking the following combination of single herbs provides a firm foundation for healing fertility. As you'll see later in the book, additional herbs will be added to address specific fertility challenges.

For women:	*For men:*
• *Red raspberry leaves*	• *Damiana*
• *Damiana*	• *Kelp*
• *Kelp*	• *Saw Palmetto*
• *Blessed thistle*	• *Gotu Kola*
• *Queen of the Meadow*	• *Zinc*

Continue this basic therapy program until achieving conception. I'll offer something more for women like Lauren who've suffered from IUD damage and undergone surgery of a perforated uterus.

To increase your healing abilities and prevent scar tissue and adhesions, use the following combination of herbs for two to three weeks after surgery:

• *Zinc*

• *Yarrow*

• *Grape Seed Extract*

In the glossary at the end of the book, you'll find detailed descriptions of these and other amazing herbs, as well as specific guidelines on dosages. For now, have faith and take heart: there is a solution to your fertility problems! Your dream of creating a tiny, precious miracle can come true.

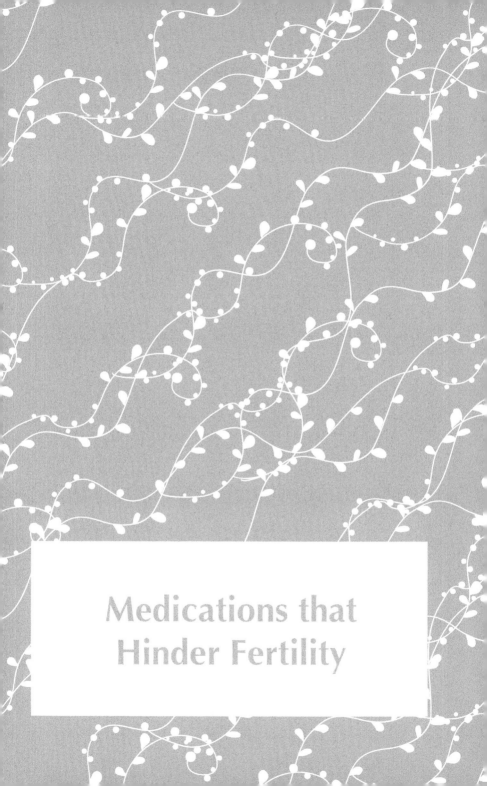

Medications that
Hinder Fertility

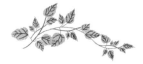

According to a recent study published in the *Journal of the American Medical Association (JAMA)*, nearly 60 percent of Americans take at least one prescription drug. Research also shows that some 80 percent of U.S. adults reach for over-the-counter medications as their first response to minor ailments. Most couples never consider pharmaceutical drugs a problem when conceiving a baby. However, most drugs prescribed today for the most common ailments, and OTC painkillers, definitely have an impact on fertility. In any fertility challenge a woman or man may be going through, the use of pharmaceutical drugs is a huge factor to consider.

Many women use painkilling NSAIDs on a monthly basis to alleviate their painful menstrual cramps. First, it is important for a woman to understand it is not normal to suffer intense pain and pelvic cramps during your menstrual period. Pain is always an indication of an underlying problem. With menstrual pain, that underlying problem is often inflammation in the pelvic area or uterus. As I also touched on earlier, when a woman gets into the habit of regularly taking NSAIDs, particularly ibuprofen, she increases her likelihood of experiencing luteinized unruptured follicle syndrome: an unfortunate condition in which eggs are never released for conception. This was the case for a patient of mine, Rachel: a woman in her mid-thirties struggling with regular, severe menstrual pain and frustrating fertility challenges.

In addition to her ibuprofen dependence, Rachel had been taking birth control pills since she was a teenager. Like many women, Rachel was prescribed birth control pills during adolescence to help manage the monthly reoccurrence of excruciating menstrual cramps. Sadly, birth control pills prescribed to "correct" this problem only mask the symptoms of the root cause: inflammation in the pelvic area. Despite the birth control remedy, Rachel still had to take ibuprofen during her menstrual cycle just so she could "function," as she put it.

Rachel and her partner wanted to have a child together. To achieve that dream, although dreading that her menstrual pain would escalate and become unbearable, she stopped taking the pill. After speaking to her gynecologist, who reassured her that her fertility would "come back," Rachel felt confident that she would be able to conceive quickly. As month after month went by with no delayed period, no relief from those terrible cramps, and no positive pregnancy test results to feel joyful about, Rachel began to seek alternative solutions to her fertility problem. In 2006, based on the referral of another patient, Rachel came to see me.

During Rachel's consultation, I determined the underlying cause of her fertility challenge: luteinized unruptured follicle (LUF) syndrome. As I explained, LUF is a failure of ovulation that occurs, according to experts, in about 10 percent of the menstrual cycles of normal, healthy, fertile women. The occurrence of LUF has been linked to unexplained infertility, endometriosis, pelvic adhesions, and the use of non-steroidal anti-inflammatory drugs—yes, NSAIDs like ibuprofen. I assured Rachel that this syndrome, which I see time and again in female patients, is an obstacle to fertility that can be overcome. As I shed light on her symptoms and explained the steps towards a solution, her face softened as I eased her mind and restored her hope in conceiving that precious baby she and her partner longed for.

I recommended that Rachel begin with the basic herbal detoxification program I shared with you. In her case, however, I recommended this not just for the two weeks I usually advise, but for four weeks. A full month of cleansing is what I felt her body needed to recover from years and years of the toxins built up from taking birth control pills daily and ibuprofen on a monthly basis.

While eager to try my natural approach to conception, Rachel again expressed her fear of the pain that would plague her come her next period. Along with her cleansing and detoxification program, I recommended a wonderful natural painkiller that also works to reduce inflammation: *Grape Seed Extract.*

I want to impress this on every reader—man or woman— who is struggling with fertility challenges. If you frequently experience pain, whether mild muscle aches or severe cramps, and use any sort of pain reliever, then seriously consider stopping these harmful drugs. For the sake of your overall health as well as your ability to achieve conception, break the habit of immediately suppressing pain with a toxic chemical pill. Instead, start listening to what pain is telling you about your body.

Pain is an alarm, a mechanism our bodies use to alert us to a problem within the body. Pain lets us know to pay attention to what the underlying cause might be. In reality, pain can truly be our body's best friend. If our bodies never felt pain, we would not be alerted that something is wrong and needs our utmost attention. Pain helps us to identify the severity, location, and type of problem we could be having so that we can treat the right area as soon as possible.

What if, like Rachel, your pain is making it extremely difficult to carry out your daily, normal tasks? Persistent, relentless pain can drain us of strength, drain our spirits, cause us to make decisions and act in ways that seem erratic and irrational, and even alter our core personality. Since humans are so afraid of pain, it is understandable why painkillers are so widely sought after and habitually used. When we no longer have pain, we can think clearly, live, and work better. The problem is that most people do not address the underlying cause of the pain. Natural therapies are much more effective than drugs and without all the harmful side effects. Herbal pain managers have much broader healing powers than analgesic drugs. Herbs that help with pain work to soothe and relieve at a deeper level. Herbal healers, like the widely trusted supplement *Grape Seed Extract* and many others, allow you not to be overwhelmed by the trauma, but to use the pain's information about your body towards healing.

For any woman who suffers every month like Rachel did, please know that taking *Grape Seed Extract* in combination with the Female Essential Herbal Fertility Program I presented will help ease menstrual pain and cramps while working to increase your fertility. Men, please also know that you can use *Grape Seed Extract* along with the Male Essential Herbal Fertility Program to find relief from your aches and pains—including testicular pain, due to inflammation of the testicles, which many men experience—while strengthening your fertility. These programs must be used by both partners until conception is achieved. I put together these combinations of herbs specifically to help strengthen overall health and the reproductive system.

Let's delve further into why taking pharmaceutical drugs hinders fertility. All chemical drugs, whether prescription medications, over-the-counter pain relievers, or narcotics, have a toxic effect on the liver. One of the body's most hardworking and crucial organs, the liver is the main filter of all chemicals ingested into the body. The powerful chemical plant of the body, the liver is the precious organ that filters out toxins at a rate of over a quart of blood per minute, when it is healthy.

The primary organ involved in filtering fat by manufacturing bile to digest fats and prevent constipation, the liver is a warehouse for minerals, vitamins, and enzymes that are released to maintain and build healthy cells. We humans depend on our liver to thrive, to procreate—to live! The liver must be healthy and strong to metabolize not only fat but also hormone excesses. The liver is key to maintaining the hormonal balance vital to achieving conception. Drugs weaken the liver and, in turn, weaken fertility.

What are the signs of a weakened liver?
Your liver may be overloaded, congested, and exhausted if you complain of or exhibit any of the following conditions:

Frequent headaches and/or migraines, and persistent, unexplained fatigue.

Allergy problems, allergic reactions (such as sinus infections), frequent cold, and flu infections.

A yellow tint to the skin or skin disorders such as psoriasis, eczema, age spots, or acne rosacea.

Bloating, digestive discomfort, or gas that becomes worse after a fatty meal. (Remember, the liver is involved in fat metabolism).

High cholesterol levels.

Chronic hepatitis or liver cirrhosis. Symptoms of liver cirrhosis include jaundice, abdominal distention (an excessively protruding stomach on a moderately thin man or woman), and increasing fatigue and weakness. Large bruises and anemia come about as cirrhosis progresses.

It bears repeating: ALL pharmaceutical drugs impact the liver and fertility. The majority of women and men in America take at least one prescription drug, and close to half of Americans take two prescription drugs. What drugs are you taking that could be aggravating your attempts to conceive a child? According to WebMD, here are the top five most common ailments among Americans today and the top five most common drugs prescribed to treat them:

Diabetes: Metformin, Actos, Januvia, Byetta, Welchol.

High cholesterol: Simvastatin, Lipitor, Crestor, Zocor, Pravastatin. (Note: these statin drugs are well-documented causing damage to the liver.)

Anxiety/Depression: Prozac, Zoloft, Cymbalta, Wellbutrin, Nardil.

Pain: Hydrocodone-Acetaminophen, Lyrica, Tramadol, Neurontin, Oxycodone.

High blood pressure: Lisinopril, Atenolol, Bystolic, Diovan, HCTZ (hydrochlorothiazide).

While we're on the topic of toxic drugs, let's go back to the story I shared earlier, the story of Lauren and Freddy. As you may recall, Freddy had suffered with epileptic seizures since childhood. From the time he was a little boy, he had been taking a prescription drug called Keppra. An anticonvulsant, Keppra is used to treat seizures. Freddy and Lauren had an inkling *that maybe this drug was at least one of the reasons they were having trouble conceiving. As I assured them, listening to your inner self is the first step on the journey to achieving conception–and, yes, Freddy and Lauren were on the right track: Keppra was, indeed, a factor in hindering their fertility.*

How could this be so? According to Drugs.com, these are some of the side effects associated with Keppra:

Infection, drowsiness, weakness, nervousness, headache, depression, agitation, aggressive behavior, fatigue, personality disorder, apathy, hyperkinesia, hostility, anxiety, mood changes, dizziness, vertigo, neck pain, chills, sore throat or hoarseness, diarrhea, dry mouth, fever, headache, hyperventilation, irregular heartbeats, joint pain, loss of appetite, lower back or side pain, muscle aches, nausea and vomiting, painful or difficult urination, paranoia, quick to react or overreact emotionally, restlessness, shaking, shivering, shortness of breath, stuffy or runny nose, sweating, trouble sleeping, irritability, and crying.

Sad, isn't it? Burdened by such side effects, how could any-one possibly think about sex, let alone enjoy making love and make a baby?

For Freddy, I recommended an herbal alternative to the toxic Keppra: *Catnip*. Yes, *Catnip* works to prevent night seizures. Freddy slept more soundly; strengthened his general health, physical fitness, and fertility; and, with Lauren, brought a precious baby son into the world.

For every couple with fertility challenges who takes any pharmaceutical drug, here's what I strongly suggest to strengthen, rebuild, and protect the liver. To the basic fertility herbal therapy program, I recommend that both women and men add the following herb: *Milk Thistle.*

If you have a medical condition for which a conventional allopathic doctor has prescribed a pharmaceutical drug, you do not have to stop taking that medication (although knowing that all drugs have so many unsettling side effects, I recommend doing all you can to eliminate pharmaceutical medications from your lifestyle regimen, whenever possible). All of these herbal combinations are safe to take along with any medication.

Now, let's move on to another common ailment today that is related to other vital organs very much involved in fertility: high blood pressure and the kidneys. In naturopathy we learn, as one of my teachers emphatically stated in one of my classes 26 years ago: "There is no such thing as high blood pressure, only weak kidneys." Fascinating, isn't it? If you or your partner suffers with this health challenge and takes a prescription drug for it, then know that the kidneys are being stimulated by a chemical diuretic and, with time, will become dependent on this chemical agent.

You may wonder: why are diuretics prescribed to control high blood pressure? Because the kidneys are directly involved in blood pressure health. Interestingly, Chinese medicine also teaches us that the kidneys are the root organs involved in the health of the female and male reproductive systems! And when a couple is having fertility challenges, the focus in Chinese medicine is directed primarily on strengthening, balancing, and rebuilding kidney health.

One of the sad side effects of pharmaceutical chemicals prescribed for high blood pressure is that they diminish sex drive, drastically, in both women and men. If a couple hardly has sexual intercourse because one partner (or both) is not "in the mood," then how can they possibly have a baby easily? This is a factor I have come across time and again with patients.

Chinese medicine teaches us that the kidneys represent the Water Element. This ancient discipline uses the following theory when it comes to describing the crucial role of the kidneys: "Water is known to nourish the roots of things, and when water flows, 'all is well,' but when water is stagnant, illness and disease can set in the body."

What if you are a woman who has blocked fallopian tubes? I bet that rings familiar with so many reading this book. When a woman has blocked fallopian tubes, impeding the egg released by the ovary from traveling to its rightful destination, Chinese medicine considers it a kidney challenge; this "block in flow" results from a stagnation of the kidneys. My success in fertility treatment stems from a strong focus on organs most would never consider.

What should you do to support fertility if you or your partner is dealing with high blood pressure, taking a prescription medical drug for this condition, and/or has a history of kidney challenges?

My recommendation is to incorporate the following herbs into your basic fertility herbal therapy program to normalize kidney activity, reduce any possible inflammation of the kidneys, control any underlying kidney infection, and cleanse and detoxify these organs to increase fertility:

- *For both men and women:* **Astragalus**
- *Additionally, for women only:* **Dong Quai**
- *Additionally, for women only who also have blocked fallopian tubes:* **Bayberry**

These herbs can be safely taken together with any high blood pressure medication you may be using. If you are seeing an allopathic, conventional doctor, then have him or her monitor your blood pressure. You will begin to start showing improvement, and soon, on your doctor's recommendation, you will be able to reduce the potency of your medication or even begin to slowly wean yourself off blood pressure drugs.

By choosing a natural healing method, regardless of your health or medical condition, use of pharmaceutical drugs, and particular fertility challenges, there is hope for achieving conception. That, above all, is what I want you to believe. I hope the stories of my experience with patients do just that! Be filled with hope as we continue our journey together. With every page you turn, you will find solutions to help your and your partner's bodies become stronger, healthier, and more open to receiving that bundle of joy you so wish for!

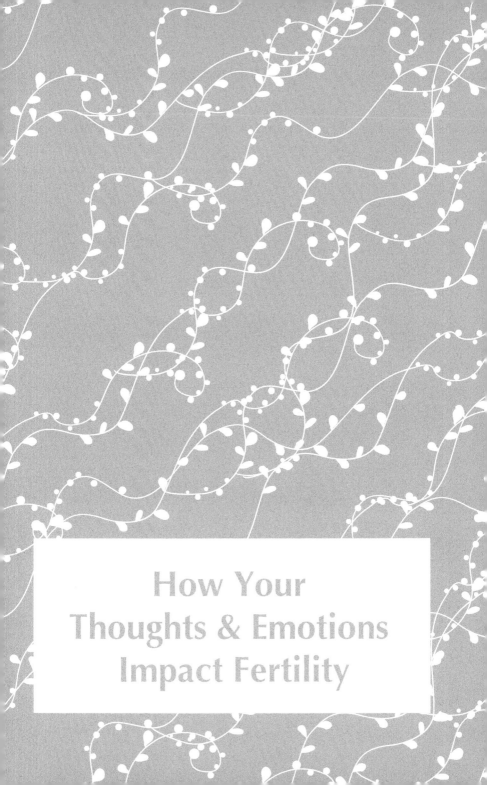

How Your
Thoughts & Emotions
Impact Fertility

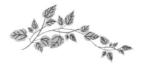

As you now know, there are many underlying causes of fertility challenges. And those causes are not limited to physical conditions. Negative thoughts and emotional turmoil often aggravate and obstruct couples' efforts to conceive. Trying and failing to get pregnant is an emotionally draining ordeal. Consider the results of two studies reported in the *Harvard Mental Health Letter.* The first, a study of 200 couples seen consecutively at a fertility clinic, found that half of the women and 15 percent of the men said that infertility was, "the most upsetting experience of their lives." The second study assessed psychological questionnaires completed by nearly 500 women. As their answers revealed, women with fertility challenges felt as anxious or depressed as those diagnosed with cancer, hypertension, or recovering from a heart attack.

If you are struggling with fertility challenges, you almost certainly will not be surprised by those findings. However, you may be surprised by the insights I am about to share with you. Thoughts and emotions can hinder fertility long before a couple begins to try to make a baby. Anger, resentment, fear, and other negative thoughts and emotions have a profound effect on the fertility of both men and the women.

In this chapter, I will share the example of one such woman, a patient of mine named Simone. When she first sought me out for help with her fertility challenges in February 2006, Simone was 40 years old. She and her husband had two beautiful children, a boy and a girl, both school age. Yet, in addition to her desire to lose weight and become healthy and fit again, Simone yearned to give birth again. She and her husband wished to have a third child. Simone had no difficulty conceiving her first two children. For this reason, she found it surprising that after months of trying, she was having difficulty conceiving. Discouraged and frustrated, feeling her age might be a factor, she came to see me with hope in her eyes.

During her consultation, I found Simone to be very healthy. Most notably, her blood pressure was ideal at 110/62. (Normal blood pressure is 120/80. At a level slightly lower than the 'norm,' Simone's blood pressure indicated that she was able to cope with stress remarkably well). Her menstrual period had always been on time every month. Yes, her weight was a factor—at 5 feet 3 inches tall, she weighed 151 pounds—but not a significant concern. I wanted to reach deeper to understand what I felt was possibly impeding her from conceiving: negative thoughts and feelings, and an emotional blockage.

During her examination, I noticed some weakness of the liver, the bladder, the right sides of both the thyroid and parathyroid, and the left ovary. Before I explain what my findings revealed about Simone's fertility challenges, I'd like to shed more light on the role of thoughts and emotions in regards to health, both generally and specifically related to the reproductive system. Our thoughts and emotions affect our bodies physically. It is very important to understand how this is so. Think about your own experience. When you dwell on sad thoughts, or feel sad, do you feel lethargic and weighed down, physically heavy? When you are thinking joyous thoughts, and feel happy, do you feel light and airy? The physical effect of thoughts and emotions is clearer in the simple example I often use with my patients. When a person imagines fearful images, feels extremely frightened and terrified, they begin to tremble, sweat profusely, and may even urinate on themselves. Now look deeper, my friends. The frightful thoughts and emotion, fear, came first, and the physical reactions came later.

Now that you understand this basic thought-emotion-body connection, open your mind to a higher level of thought. Within holistic medicine and Chinese medicine, there are many teachings that affirm the connection between 'specific' organs and 'specific' thoughts and emotions.

Holistic medicine teaches us how thoughts and emotions affect the physical body in the following manner:

Consciousness. *To be in a state of consciousness affects the skin and the hypothalamus. It is expressed through consciously feeling and expressing enthusiasm and strong, confident, positive statements one thinks or says such as: "I am..." "I see..." "I feel..." "I choose..." "I know..." "I enjoy..." and "I love..."*

Unresolved Forgiveness. *This negative thought, not forgiving others, or not forgiving oneself, affects the kidneys and bladder. People bogged down by this thought are thin-skinned and cling to resentment. It is expressed through statements such as: "I will never forget what you did to hurt me." "Though* it happened ten years ago, I still feel the sting." "That is still a very sensitive subject." "Your behavior was inexcusable."

Not Letting Go. This negative thought affects the colon/large intestine. Those who feel they must be in control all the time, in control of other people, and of every circumstance and situation carry this thought. When a person nags frequently, continuously harps on the same thing, over and over again, or micromanages, he or she is "not letting go."

Pain. This thought and feeling affects the hypothalamus. When people are dealing with feeling hurt, feeling as if their spirit and soul are in pain in response to loss, betrayal, etc., their entire body might feel achy, or specific targeted areas could be hurting with no real explanation for the existing pain. Statements and thoughts that express pain include: "My suffering feels unbearable." "The misery seems endless." "Why did you do this to me? It hurts so much."

Anger. This emotion affects the liver, the gallbladder, the thyroid, and the parathyroid. The liver and gallbladder are affected by internal anger or rage. The thyroid and parathyroid are affected by verbal anger. Verbal anger can be silent; when someone "chokes themself" on bitterness or "swallows" their anger. On the opposite end of the spectrum, verbal anger can be expressed quite vocally—by someone who is cursing, yelling, screaming, ranting, and/or raving. Or, in many cases, a person harboring verbal anger exhibits both extremes. Statements that express verbal anger include: "I hate that!" "I hate you!" "How dare you!" "I'll get even!" "You can't make me!

Unconsciousness. Negative unconscious thoughts affect the ovaries and testicles. These thoughts are expressed by people who avoid feeling too deeply, avoid getting too attached, or have problems trusting others, most times because they are afraid of getting hurt or of getting hurt again. Imagine a person overwhelmed by life's blows, who feels as if blocking their emotions will protect them from continued despair. Imagine this person, in an effort to drown out their life's problems, consuming excessive amounts of alcohol and then passing out on the sofa, the empty glass falling from their hand and rolling slowly onto the floor, all this so they no longer have to 'feel' or a person who uses illegal substances or chemical agents to get 'high' so they can escape the real world around them so they don't have to 'feel' the misery they are living. A person like this, who has decided to numb their feelings, is exhibiting unconsciousness. Statements include: "I don't know." "I don't care." "I don't understand." "Just leave me alone." I don't want to feel..."

Chinese medicine teaches us how thoughts and emotions affect the physical body in the following manner:

* *Anger emotion affects the liver.*
* *Dissatisfaction and feeling 'burnt-out' affects the heart.*
* *Worrying constantly and nervousness affect the spleen-pancreas meridian.*
* *Defensiveness and grief affect the lungs and respiratory system.*
* *Fear affects the kidneys and bladder.*

Now that you have a broad understanding of how thoughts, feelings and emotions affect physical health, let's focus on how thoughts and emotions specifically affect the reproductive system of women and men to interfere with fertility. When working with couples who so desperately want to have a baby together and are having trouble conceiving, I incorporate the knowledge from both holistic medicine and Chinese

*medicine to address four specific feelings and emotions that I
have found are the most relevant to fertility:*

1. Anger / verbal anger (liver, thyroid, and parathyroid)

2. Unresolved forgiveness (kidneys and bladder)

3. Fear (kidneys)

4. Unconsciousness (ovaries and testicles)

Now, let's go back to Simone's story. As you may recall,
I found weaknesses and imbalances in some of Simone's
organs: the liver, bladder, the right side of the thyroid and
parathyroid, and left ovary. From these findings, as I told
Simone, I had a strong hunch that she was dealing with
some anger, unresolved forgiveness, and unconsciousness
issues. She asked me to explain further what I meant.

What I shared with Simone drew on trusted theories in naturopathy and holistic medicine. As I learned many years
ago, the left side of the body represents the feminine aspect
of the body. We are taught that challenges on this side of
the body are related to: female figures in one's life (could
also be in relation to oneself if the person with the health
challenge is a woman), and worry or concern about their
survival in love and emotional relationships. The right side
of the body, as naturopathy and holistic medicine teaches,
represents the masculine aspect of the body.

Challenges on this side of the body are related to: masculine
figures in one's life (again could also be in relation to oneself if the person with the said health challenge is a man),
and also deals with worry or concern about their survival in

the form of financial matters, business relationships, work issues, educational matters, and career matters.

What was Simone's body telling me? The liver is affected negatively by the emotion of anger. The bladder is affected negatively by the emotion of unresolved forgiveness. The thyroid and parathyroid are affected negatively by anger and, specifically, verbal anger. I explained to Simone that I had a hunch she was dealing with some anger and unresolved forgiveness issues towards a male figure.

Simone stared at me in awe. After a few moments of silence, she began to tell me how, after their second child, she had discovered her husband had been unfaithful to her—with a woman who worked for her at the time.

I compassionately listened to her story. As you will find when you visit a naturopathic doctor, we take the time to truly listen to our patients. I feel this is so very crucial to the work I do and contributes so very much to the healing of my patients and clients. When Simone was done sharing her sad experience of betrayal, how she held her anger towards him inside and still had not truly forgiven him while putting on a smile for the world outside, I explained to her how this very harboring of negative thoughts and emotions was what was hindering her from conceiving the third baby she so wanted.

Now, you may be asking, well, what about the weakness of the left ovary? The ovaries are affected negatively by unconsciousness, or blocking one's feelings towards others. I continued to explain that I also had a hunch she was dealing with unconsciousness thought/emotion, and 'blocking' a female figure emotionally. She explained the woman who worked for her, the woman her husband was unfaithful with, used to be a long-time friend of hers. What's more, she had recently found out that the twins this woman had given birth to were her husband's children.

Although this story is heartbreaking, it is very common. Could you be a couple that is dealing with similar emotional turmoil? I am sure many of you can relate to this. Although Simone was rebuilding her marriage and felt a strong desire, as her husband did, to have another child together, she was holding these negative emotions in, harboring them to the point that they were affecting her body physically.

How was Simone to overcome these feelings to increase her chances of conceiving a baby? I explained she needed to forgive her husband and release the blockage of emotion towards the woman with whom he was unfaithful. She understood. As we continued our discussion, I recommended Simone write her husband a letter. She was not to let him know she was doing so, but to carry this task out, peacefully, on her own. I urged her to take the time after her consultation with me that day to find a quiet, peaceful place to sit comfortably and begin writing the letter. I recommended her first sentence state, "I am not doing this for you; I am doing this for me." This first sentence of the forgiveness letter is so very important. It sets the stage so that from the very beginning, the reader understands that what they are about to read is not necessarily an attack on them, but a true focus on the writer and their feelings. Then, she was to proceed by detailing everything he did and failed to do that angered her from the moment they met before the beginning of the marriage, what hurt her, what bothered her—everything, up until that point in time.

All the negative thoughts, feelings, and emotions she felt towards her husband needed to be expressed handwritten, pulled from her inner being to the sheets of paper with every stroke of her pen. (Note: In today's day and age, very few people take the time to write with a writing utensil and piece of paper. Most writing is done through emails, texts, etc., and it is crucial to understand that a forgiveness letter process does not initiate healing within the writer if it is written in this 'technical' manner. When one writes what one is thinking and feeling by hand, it is as if the emotions, whether they be negative or positive ones, within the writer are coming forth, brought out of the subconscious mind to be released with every stroke of their pen, and felt by the reader as they read every single letter. This is powerful for healing from within.)

At the end of this letter, after she has written absolutely everything and expressed exactly how she feels, I explained that in the last paragraph she must write that she forgives her husband. After she forgives him, she should then write within the same paragraph that she asks him to forgive her for ever having any resentments towards him. That is all she was to say on her behalf, no matter what else might have transpired between them in the trajectory of their long relationship.

I further advised Simone that she was to not 'prepare' him by telling him that a letter was being written, that she was not to be there when he read the letter, and not to expect a response after writing it. After writing the letter, she was then instructed to let him know she wrote him a letter, tell him where she left it for him to find, then to proceed with her day.

This process is a tool I was taught to use during my naturopathy studies over 26 years ago. Naturopathic doctors recommend this so patients are able to overcome negative thoughts and emotions we know are affecting them physically.

It is a must, a necessary action that must be taken against anger, unresolved forgiveness, fear, unconsciousness, and all negative thoughts and emotions that could be affecting the body physically. This is a weight that must be lifted from a person's spirit so one can be 'open to receive' baby, clear the house that is the body and achieve inner peace to allow conception.

I recommend the herb *Milk Thistle* for strengthening the liver, an organ that, as you already know, is crucial to fertility. When taking this herb, be comforted as the feelings of inner anger and rage are dispelled. As the body and mind are so connected, seeing this process unfold is truly fascinating and remarkable. For the kidneys, I recommend herbs such as *Astragalus* for both men and women and *Dong Quai* for women only. With these herbs, the kidneys—the root of the health of the reproductive system—become balanced and unresolved forgiveness issues are slowly overcome.

Simone's verbal anger, indicated by the weakened right side of her thyroid and parathyroid, stemmed from not talking to her husband when she was outraged by his infidelity and instead 'choking herself' from expressing her feelings. This was also something we needed to address. To do this, I recommended she use the Female Essential Fertility Herbal Therapy program, which contains the following herb, rich in natural iodine and known for nourishing the thyroid gland: *Kelp.*

As I emphatically expressed, this process needed to be done. Simone agreed and promised to carry it out. Now you may be asking yourselves, how could this be done so easily? You may be a couple reading this who, even if you're not dealing with the same situation, may be harboring negative thoughts and emotions such as these and find it hard to just 'let them go.' Please know, my dear readers, that as I stated earlier, when one strengthens a weakened organ, the negative emotions related to that organ dissipate very easily. Healing from these hurtful thoughts, feelings, and emotions is not difficult once you are utilizing the herbal solutions that strengthen and fortify the organs involved.

The link between the thyroid and fertility challenges is supported by research in conventional allopathic medicine, as well as naturopathy, holistic medicine, and Chinese medicine. To quote fertility experts at the Mayo Clinic: "There is sometimes a link between hypothyroidism—when you have an underactive thyroid gland—and infertility in women. With hypothyroidism, your thyroid gland doesn't produce enough of certain important hormones. Low levels of thyroid hormone can interfere with the release of an egg from your ovary (ovulation), which impairs fertility. In addition, some of the underlying causes of hypothyroidism— such as certain autoimmune or pituitary disorders—may impair fertility. For women, treating hypothyroidism is an important part of any effort to correct infertility..."

Simone also had to confront her unconsciousness thoughts/emotions toward the woman with whom her husband had twins. As I mentioned, holding on to unconsciousness is as if one has built an emotional wall to block one's feelings, and it directly affects a woman's ovaries and a man's testicles. Since this wall that the person has created is directly related to the reproductive system, the body then can become prone to creating a wall of abnormal cells. This presence of abnormal cells can show up as cysts, polyps, or tumors. In a woman, unconsciousness could make her more prone to developing uterine fibroids or endometriosis, breast cysts, ovarian cysts, tumors on the ovaries, or blocked fallopian tubes. These 'abnormal cell walls' that may develop within the body as a result of holding on to unconsciousness thoughts are a wall the body creates to prevent anyone from penetrating that person emotionally. For Simone, the Female Essential Herbal Fertility Program already contains an herb, which nourishes the ovaries: *Red Raspberry*. For men grappling with unconsciousness thoughts, within the Male Essential Herbal Fertility Program is the following potent healing herb which strengthens the testes, given testicles make male hormones, including testosterone, and produce sperm, all necessary aspects to a man's fertility: *Saw Palmetto*.

Building up an emotional wall is so detrimental to the well-being of the reproductive system. Tear it down! You deserve to feel you can open up to, share your love, and care for anyone who is in your life! If you feel like hugging a person to demonstrate your love, do so; if you feel like kissing that person, do so; if you feel like shouting from the mountain top how much you love a person, do so! Holding back from expressing your feelings does not only hurt the other person. It directly hurts you. And it directly hurts your ability to achieve conception.

Fortunately, Simone's sad story of betrayal, negative emotions, and fertility problems has a happy ending! Eight months after committing to and continuing to follow my recommended herbal therapy program, Simone became pregnant with her third child, a gorgeous baby boy. Two years later, in July 2008, she unexpectedly became pregnant with her fourth child, another boy. As I am also delighted to report, Simone and her husband moved beyond anger and resentment before she became pregnant after she wrote her letter, and her husband finally understood her deep feelings and now truly feels she has forgiven him. They have a strong, loving marriage today and are loving parents to four children.

Simone did not experience one of the four negative thoughts and emotions that affect fertility: Fear. That emotion, as Chinese medicine teaches, is directly related to kidney health. I have found many times working with patients that the underlying fear of the unknown, especially if they were trying to conceive their first child, was something a couple had to overcome to truly help their bodies be 'open to receive' conception. Fear about how their lives will change, fear of who would take care of the child once the mother goes back to work, etc., are some of the fears numerous couples have shared with me over the years.

If you are a couple who feels there may be some fear issues you are both dealing with, I have already shared the ideal herbs for strengthening the kidneys and overcoming fears: *Astragalus* and, additionally for women, *Dong Quai.* All negative thoughts and emotions cause "clutter" within the body. Your thoughts, feelings, and emotions must be in balance and free flowing to have strong reproductive systems. The solutions are here for you to achieve the balance between the body and mind necessary to conceive a child.

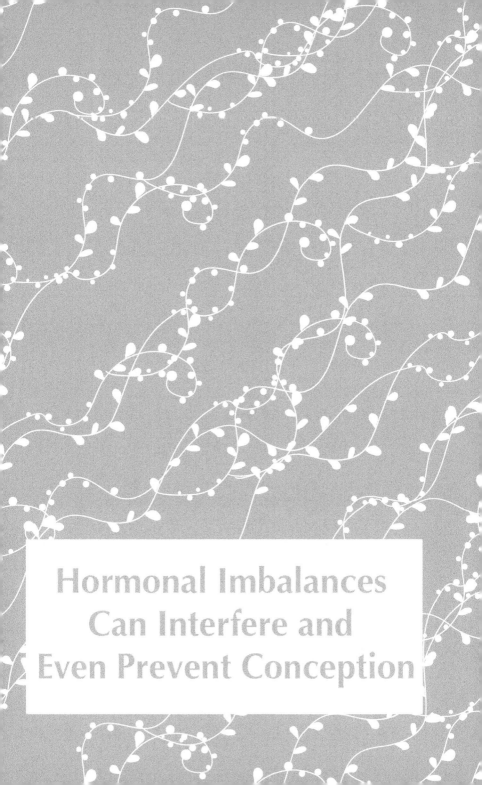

Hormonal Imbalances
Can Interfere and
Even Prevent Conception

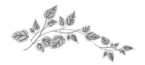

B alanced hormones in men and women are necessary to conceive a child. Research has found that environmental hormone mimics from chemicals and pollutants, like xenoestrogens found in styrofoam products, are very much linked to infertility in both men and women. That means your hormones in general must be balanced if you are to conceive child. Let us begin by discussing hormone imbalances in women.

Women — yes, even strong women— are such delicate beings with intricate systems. Nature shows how a woman's body works in a lovely, complex balance. A woman should be able to rejoice in her very essence, feel marvelous, and love her body, but the many intricacies of her system are precisely tuned. Shifts in her inner balance can throw her hormones out of sync, causing extreme reactions, positive and negative.

From the time a woman has her first menstrual period through her childbearing years to the 'change of life' called pre-menopause, full menopause, and, finally, post-menopause, many women today are blasted with hormonal shifts that disrupt their lives.

Based on data quoted in the *New England Journal of Medicine*, as many as 10 percent of women of childbearing age— some 6 million women in the U.S.— have polycystic ovary syndrome. PCOS is a hormone imbalance problem that can interfere with normal ovulation.

Its cause is unknown, but it is the most common hormonal abnormality in reproductive age women and a principal cause of female infertility. From puberty through middle age and beyond, hormones regulate just about everything in women from how we feel emotionally and physically to our energy level, from our regular monthly period to challenges with swelling and inflammation. Hormonal imbalance is a root factor in many female health problems including: headaches and migraines (associated with nausea and vomiting), depression, premenstrual syndrome (PMS), uterine fibroids, endometriosis, low libido (low sexual desire), and, of course, infertility.

With all the hormones found in animal protein, meats, genetically modified organisms (GMOs), pesticides, chemicals, combined with all the toxic, harmful substances we are exposed to today, it is difficult to maintain hormonal balance. We are literally bombarded with man-made hormones, like the worldwide and widespread hormone-mimicking chemicals and pollutants, hormones injected in food, and chemical hormone drugs.

A lifestyle marked by high stress doesn't help either. Certain lifestyle changes can make a great impact on helping the body become hormonally harmonized. There is truly no need for any woman to turn to a drug to balance her hormones after prolonged stress, traumas, or a severe illness.

Drugs have many unpleasant side effects, including the risk of stopping natural hormone production completely. Natural herbal hormonal balancing therapies help the body to achieve its very own healthy hormone levels and restore true inner balance.

How, you might be wondering, would a woman know if her hormones are out of balance? Signals from a woman's body that hormonal imbalance could be a problem include:

- *Spotting between menstrual cycles*
- *Mood swings, irritability, melancholy feelings, and depression*
- *Frequent water retention*
- *Severe menstrual discomfort every month, painful periods, intermittent periods, or lack of periods*
- *And, as I mentioned earlier, reproductive system challenges such as uterine fibroids, endometriosis, and PCOS.*

Knowing that PCOS is one of the most prevalent hormonal imbalances that causes infertility in women, I'd like to share the story of a woman who suffered from—and overcame—this condition. Her name is Malina. In 2013, Mina, Malina's older sister and a patient of mine for over 7 years, came in for one of her follow up appointments. During the course of our conversation, Mina confided her little sister's health problem to me.

Mina's sister, Malina, was 24 years old. Mina explained that for years her dear sister was suffering with extremely heavy periods, lack of periods, bloating, weight gain, and excessive facial hair. Plagued by these problems, Malina sought out a gynecologist four years earlier. Malina was told she had severe PCOS. But that wasn't the only distressing news from her doctor. Malina was also told she was infertile. Imagine it: learning you are infertile at the young age of 20. Mina explained her little sister was heartbroken, as was the rest of their family. With no real solution for her PCOS problem and accepting that she would never be able to get pregnant naturally, Malina had been having unprotected sex. She now longed to conceive a child with the man she loved, her partner for the past few years, yet believed that was impossible.

Mina was desperate to help Malina find relief from PCOS and fulfill her dream of becoming a mother. I shared with Mina the very same Female Essential Fertility Herbal Therapy Program I shared with all of you. In addition, I prescribed one specific Brazilian herb that has the amazing properties to help with cysts in the body: *Pau D'arco.*

Mina purchased all the recommended herbs for her sister. Eager to try a natural remedy, Malina followed my recommendations consistently. Less than two months after, Mina received the amazing, joyful news that she would soon be an aunt for the first time. Malina conceived naturally and gave birth to a gorgeous, sassy little girl. Her 'princess' is now 18 months old.

If you are a woman frustrated by failed attempts to conceive, could the problem be PCOS? Let's delve a bit more into this female health challenge rooted in hormonal imbalance. Women suffering with ovarian cysts are being diagnosed in increasingly high numbers. This source of discomfort is common among women with menstrual problems, whether lack of periods or irregular periods or excessive bleeding during their periods.

Do you know what ovarian cysts are? These cysts are non-malignant, small, chambered sacs that tend to be filled with fluid. Based on the latest published statistics at WomensHealth.gov:

Between 1 in 10 and 1 in 20 women of childbearing age have ovarian cysts. As many as 5 million women in the United States may be affected. It can occur in girls as young as 11 years old.

Astounding, is it not? Women who suffer with ovarian cysts do not ovulate normally, but despite pain and some fertility difficulties can still conceive. PCOS, on the other hand, is a more severe syndrome than simply ovarian cysts and leads to infertility. Ovarian cysts are most definitely hormone-driven, usually from estrogen dominance (too much estrogen) and hypothyroidism. Do you see the correlation here again between the focus on the liver and the thyroid and increasing fertility?

When overloaded with toxins, the liver cannot effectively filter hormones, which can result in estrogen dominance in women. The thyroid is also directly involved in hormonal balance; when it is low functioning—a condition called hypothyroidism — this can affect fertility.

It is important to note that ovarian cysts, which tend to stop growing after menstruation stops and menopause sets in, are not linked to cancer. However, they are very painful. Ovarian cysts cause women to feel pain, often repeatedly and intensely, during intercourse. These cysts can also provoke heavy menstrual bleeding and spotting between periods.

Polycystic ovary syndrome (PCOS) is much more severe than having one ovarian cyst or even a few cysts. This syndrome is defined by multiple cysts that develop on both ovaries causing the menstrual period to become very irregular. Symptoms associated with PCOS include:

- Insulin resistance
- Obesity
- Excessive facial hair
- Adult acne (many times acne not just on the face, but also very common on the back, chest, bumps on the upper arms, and bumps on the thighs)
- Infertility

Two very common factors in PCOS development are high chronic stress and eating disorders. There are hazards to conventional medical treatment of ovarian cysts such as hormone therapy or removal of the ovaries altogether. Along with lifestyle and dietary changes, natural hormone balancing herbs offer promise for recovering from this hormonal imbalance syndrome and overcoming fertility challenges.

How do you know if you have ovarian cysts? Warning signs include:

Severe uterine bleeding due to endometrial hyperplasia, a condition that occurs when the endometrium or lining of the uterus becomes too thick, which is directly caused by unbalanced estrogen dominance.

Chronic, severe, acute pain and/or swelling and inflammation of the fallopian tubes or ovaries, and usually, the inability to conceive a child.

Painful sexual intercourse, swollen breasts, and heel pain. (Consult any reflexology chart and you'll see: the heel is linked to reproductive health!)

Erratic menstrual cycles accompanied by pain that is difficult to pinpoint, discomfort in the breasts and lower abdomen, and unusual swelling.

Unusual weight gain (usually more upper body weight gain) due to low thyroid activity.

Unusual fevers, abdominal gas, and a coated tongue.

Excess bodily hair growth because of an imbalance between progesterone, testosterone and estrogen levels.

Now, you have an idea of how ovarian cysts and PCOS can hinder a woman's reproductive health and sexual pleasure. But what causes these unfortunate ovarian cysts? The list is long!

Consider these facts:

Estrogen dominance is the most common cause of cysts. (Remember, hormones, hormones, hormones...)

Having frequent X-rays and radiation treatments that a person undergoes for other health problems may change your cell structure and cause an environment to develop for ovarian cyst growth

Research has now pointed to long-term use of synthetic hormone replacement and birth control pills because they disrupt hormone balance

Diabetes is a major factor involved in the development of ovarian cysts, especially alcohol-induced diabetes

Unhealthy lifestyle habits, especially eating a diet high in fat and ingesting too much caffeine (toxic caffeine)

Formerly having used or currently using an IUD may also be a factor involved in the development of this syndrome

A high stress lifestyle that, in turn, causes constipation, poor elimination of wastes, and a highly acidic body, encouraging a body chemistry that becomes unhealthy and prone to developing cysts

Fortunately, recovering from ovarian cysts and PCOS and restoring fertility is possible as the story of Malina, who is now enjoying a giggly 18 month old baby girl today, affirms. My dear readers, please have faith in your body's ability to heal with the help of my natural recommendations so that you can become ready to conceive a healthy, feisty baby of your very own.

Now let's move on to the men, who have their own hormonal problems. Men, let's talk testosterone. Testosterone is absolutely essential for sperm production. I have already touched on one of the causes of fertility challenges in men: low sperm count. If a man desires to get his partner pregnant, he must have a normal sperm count and, of course, healthy sperm. The only way a man can get ample, robust sperm is if his hormones are balanced and levels of testosterone are up to par.

Unfortunately, low testosterone levels and hormonal imbalances plague many men today. Based on recent research by New England Research Institute scientists, one out of four men over 30 has low testosterone levels. And yet, according to another survey by Roper Starch Worldwide of 1,000 men, 68 percent could not name one single symptom or condition that is associated with low testosterone. Of that 68 percent, 15 percent mentioned low libido as a symptom of suffering with low testosterone. Lethargy and fatigue was named by 6 percent; low muscle mass and/or a decrease in muscle mass/muscle development was named by 3 percent; and less than one percent suggested a link between men's osteoporosis and low testosterone.

Apparently, many men lack a clear understanding of what hormones are all about and are in the dark about how hormonal imbalances drastically affect their health. One reason for this is that men's hormonal challenges have been much less researched and publicized than women's hormonal problems. Yet the fact remains: hormonal disruptions affect a man's life and fertility as much as they do a woman's.

In my practice, I have come to know many men who listen to their bodies and notice their hormonal fluctuations. I have had some men share that they can 'feel' when their partner is about to get her menstrual cycle and, further, are attuned to her because they also experience monthly changes in how they feel with irritability, melancholy, lower energy levels, impacted work performance and performance during sports activities. Keep in mind, this is not only what they feel because their partner is about to get her period. They know their bodies are going through something. They feel these hormonal shifts within their own bodies, on a monthly basis, regardless of what their partner is going through. They attribute it to the equivalent of their own monthly 'period' cycle.

What are normal testosterone levels? Normal testosterone levels in healthy men range from about 300 nanograms per deciliter (ng/dL) up to 1,000 nanograms per deciliter (ng/dL). At different times in a man's life, blood levels of testosterone can fluctuate and drastically range from 250 to 1,200 nanograms.

These shifts affect men in many ways from their endurance and vitality to their work and activity performance, to their mood and sexual performance. Yes, a man's hormonal shifts and fluctuations are not as dramatic as a woman's.

However, for those men over age 40 who wish to have a baby with their partner and are having fertility challenges, understand that testosterone levels start to decline around this age and typically continually fall, up to 10 percent every 10 years.

Plainly stated: if a man wants to increase his fertility, his hormones must be balanced and his testosterone levels must be within normal range to produce healthy sperm to achieve conception of a baby.

What symptoms let a man know his hormones are out of balance? Men, pay attention if you are experiencing the following:

- *Reduced libido (reduced sex drive)*
- *A belly with a pouch (poor abdominal muscle tone)*
- *Dribble or poor urinary control with prostate inflammation and pain*

If you or your partner are suffering from these symptoms, you should be aware of the underlying causes of hormonal imbalances in men that could be affecting your ability to conceive. Causes of male hormone problems range from:

- *Nutrient deficiencies—from drastic, severe dieting, exaggerated body building, suffering from a long illness, or recently undergoing surgery and deficiencies in calcium, protein, and iodine. (Remember, the thyroid is involved here. Iodine deficiency can cause hypothyroidism, which is linked to fertility problems in both men and women)*

- *Use of synthetic steroids*

- *Chronic stress!*

If you are a man having fertility challenges and know your testosterone levels are low, take heart: there is a solution. Let me tell you the short story of Faith and Yamin.

Faith and Yamin came to see me to help them with their fertility in July of 2006. This beautiful married couple from South Africa had been trying to conceive for many months with no hope. Faith was in her late twenties; Yamin in his early thirties.

During our consultation, they shared with me that after all the tests done with their respective doctors, Faith showed all the positive signs of being able to conceive, while Yamin's test results showed his testosterone levels were low and his sperm count was under 10 million. Yamin's problem, his conventional doctor determined, was the reason Faith could not pregnant.

The main focus in this case then was to balance Yamin's hormones and increase his testosterone levels and sperm count. However, although Faith was told she was healthy and should have no problem conceiving, I recommended they both begin their respective Essential Fertility Herbal programs. Yes, gentlemen, in your respective Male Fertility Program, the combination of two herbs and a mineral: *Saw Palmetto, Kelp,* and, *Zinc,* is going to help balance your hormones, especially testosterone.

Because low sperm count was also a challenge for Yamin, I felt the need to add the following herb—which is naturally loaded with many nutrients, including an extra boost of *Zinc*—to strengthen Yamin's fertility: *Pumpkin Seed Extract.*

Upon Faith and Yamin's follow-up visit, just a month after their initial start, we agreed they try to conceive next month. To all our joy, Faith became pregnant that month. But that is not all... Faith and Yamin are now the happy parents of twins: a boy and girl!

This is the only couple I have ever treated in 21 years who has conceived twins. Oh, but what a joy it was to hear such news! And to know this was actually Faith and Yamin's very wish was an additional blessing.

It is important to understand that the result with Faith and Yamin was specifically because of their genetic tendencies. Twins run in both their families. If this happens to be the case with you and your partner, there is always a possibility that you could conceive twins, triplets, or more. By trusting and following The Naturopathic Approach to Fertility, please be open to allowing nature to take its course. Allow your bodies to heal as we feed them what they need to become fertile vessels while allowing your spirits to be open to receive the miracle of a baby you deserve.

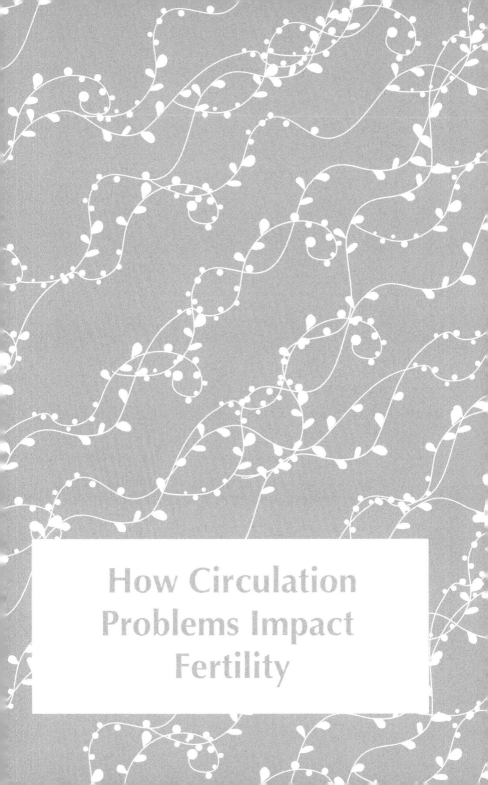

How Circulation Problems Impact Fertility

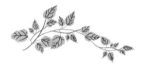

Our circulatory system health is vital. The circulatory system is made up of the blood vessels that run through the entire body. This is the river that flows throughout our bodies: a river that feeds our very existence, a river of life. The arteries carry blood away from the heart and the veins carry blood back to the heart. This river carries toxins and waste to the elimination channels of the body. Heat is transported from the interior of the body to the skin.

The circulatory system keeps us energized and alert by providing blood supply to the brain. It treats infections by carrying antibodies to the infected site. And most importantly, this is the system within the body that carries oxygen and vital nutrients to all the cells and organs.

How does this information relate to fertility? If the reproductive system is not receiving adequate blood flow with needed nutrients and oxygen to be strong and healthy, then conception is hindered. Remember I shared with you how a problem such as severe anemia should be addressed prior to conception? Anemia that results in nutritional deficiency directly affects the circulatory system.

Medical research has confirmed the link between severe anemia and fertility problems. As an article in *The Journal of the American Board of Family Medicine* states: "Though rarely encountered in women of childbearing age, untreated pernicious anemia has been found to be a cause of infertility. Once treated, conception often occurs within months."

The symptoms of anemia include: numbness and tingling of the extremities, overall weakness, yellowing of the skin, and gastrointestinal disturbances that cause a sore tongue. The condition is often marked by a partial loss of coordination of the legs, fingers, and feet. A loss of appetite along with diarrhea may also be present. In addition, nerve deterioration is known to occur.

The primary cause of pernicious anemia is a deficiency of vitamin B12.

Do you have an idea of how many people suffer with anemia? The American Society of Hematology confirms that anemia is the most common blood disorder in the U.S. today. According to the National Heart, Lung, and Blood Institute, anemia affects more than 3 million Americans.

It is crucial to have a strong circulatory system to increase fertility in both men and women. Anemia causes a weakened circulatory system. Could you or your partner be suffering with circulatory problems? Do you even know the signs to look for that indicate this condition? First, it is important to note that a sedentary lifestyle will impede proper circulatory blood flow.

Questions you should ask yourselves to determine if you could be suffering with the beginning stages of a circulatory problem are:

• *Do your feet, hands, ears, and face become chilled and cold easily?*

• *Have your ears been ringing lately?*

• *Have you been noticing memory problems?*

• *If you have answered yes to any of these questions, then your circulatory system is weak. It must be strengthened to increase fertility.*

A sluggish blood flow is an early indicator of truly serious disorders that can lead to high cholesterol, arteriosclerosis (hardening of the arteries, one of the main causes of poor erections and impotence in men), high blood pressure, phlebitis (inflammation of the vein walls), and heart disease. It can also bring on the following circulatory problems, all of which impede fertility:

Raynaud's Disease. Men, be aware of the symptoms of Raynaud's disease, known as the underlying result of atherosclerosis. Research by the Mayo Clinic states that the cause of this disease is not completely understood, and may develop unexpectedly. However, one known cause is using a chainsaw or jackhammer over a long period, several years.

Symptoms include extreme sensitivity to the cold, even when the weather is quite warm; numbness and/or a pins-and-needles sensation in the hands and feet, which often drain of color and look white. These all stem from blood flow being cut off by small arteries that contract.

Chilblains, which are characterized by itchy, very painful patches that develop on the feet and hands. Claudication, which is one of the peripheral artery diseases. Claudication is characterized by severe pain in the legs as a result of obstructed blood flow. What aggravates this disease? A low fiber diet, lack of exercise, and poor elimination of waste (constipation) are all related to claudication.

Spider Veins. These red, thin, unattractive lines that may develop on the upper arms, thighs, and the face (most times on the nose and cheeks). They are usually accompanied by muscle cramps in the legs.

Varicose Veins, which is a very common peripheral vascular circulatory problem. For many women—and some men—varicose veins are not only extremely uncomfortable but also unsightly; they are a costly cosmetic problem. Varicose veins are the direct result of leaky valves. Most times, they cause pain, cramping, lethargy, heaviness, and ankle and leg swelling. They develop when a defect in the wall of the vein dilates the vein and in turn damages the valves of the vein.

Next, when the valves of the vein do not function properly, there is an increase in blood pressure, which then results in bulging. Many times, very dangerous blood clots can develop in the veins. Inflammation of the veins, known as vasculitis, overwhelmingly afflicts women. Women suffer with vein fragility problems four times more frequently than men due to a loss of tissue tone, weakening of the vein walls, and vein fragility increases.

Signs that you may have varicose veins are:

- A tight, heavy feeling in the legs
- Painful, distended-looking leg veins
- Tingling and numbness in the legs

Causes of varicose veins are:

- A diet high in fried foods, red meat, dairy foods

- A diet low in fiber and fundamental nutrients. Lack of essential fatty acids (EFAs) and vitamins A, C, and E weakens connective tissue; as a result, weakness of the vascular wall sets in.

- Poor, weak posture

- Long periods of sitting, lifting heavy objects, or standing

This last cause— the most common cause of varicose veins— was the very reason a patient of mine, Ida, suffered with varicose and spider veins as well as fertility challenges. For more than a year prior to coming to see me, Ida had been trying to conceive a baby with no positive outcome. That soon changed after we met.

In February 2010, Ida sought me out to help her with her fertility. She was 30 years old at the time. Ida was told by her conventional doctor that she was ovulating properly, that her uterus looked healthy, and that she should have no problem conceiving. However, Ida had suffered with severe anemia for years. To aggravate matters, she was on her feet for long hours because of her demanding job as the manager of a coffee and tea shop and had developed many unsightly spider and varicose veins.

Immediately, I understood that Ida's circulatory problems were the underlying cause of her fertility problems. For over a year, she had been trying to get pregnant with her partner, who was in his late twenties and found by his urologist to be healthy.

Conventional doctors couldn't find a reason why they could

not get pregnant. Therefore, I had to be sure we focused on promoting healthy circulatory blood flow to ensure that Ida's reproductive system was being nourished properly and also to ensure that when she did conceive vital nutrients would flow through her body to the baby.

Along with her Essential Female Fertility Herbal Program, I added two herbs to feed her body natural iron and raise her red blood cell count.

These herbs would work to correct the challenge of anemia, reduce inflammation of the vein walls, strengthen vascular fragility, reduce the feeling of lethargy and heaviness, reduce pain in her legs, and stimulate blood flow throughout the body, while ensuring her reproductive organs were being nourished and receiving proper oxygen. Please note, these two following herbs are ideal for men also:

* Alfalfa
* Butcher's Broom

Four months later, in June of 2010, Ida called to tell me she was pregnant! In March of 2011, she gave birth to a handsome, smiling baby boy named Jadin. As a guest at her baby shower, I shed a few tears as she explained to her family how we worked together to help her finally feel complete.

I was honored and deeply touched by her thoughtful words of thanks and overjoyed to celebrate the imminent arrival of her baby. My dear readers, while I do not expect to be invited to your baby shower (my calendar would be overflowing!), I look forward to celebrating the imminent arrival of your baby someday soon!

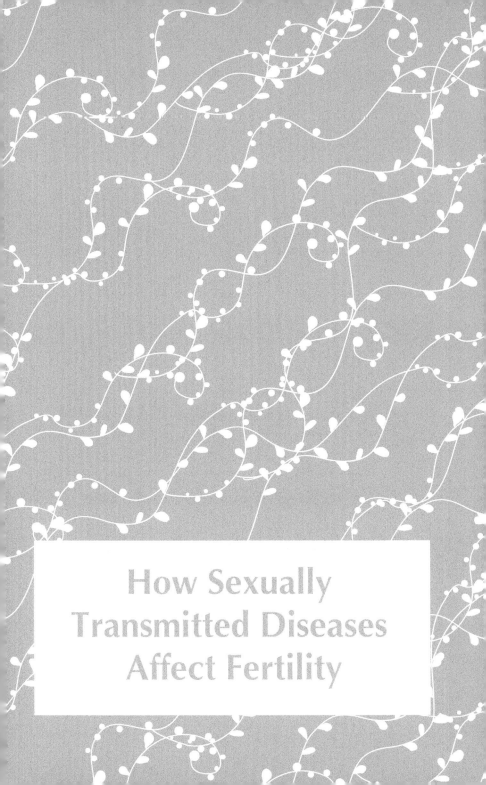

How Sexually
Transmitted Diseases
Affect Fertility

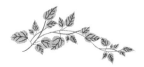

Sexually transmitted diseases (STDs) are very prevalent in today's day and age. Apart from the fact they can be traumatizing for most, STDs are a factor to consider if a couple is having problems conceiving a child. As anyone who has been infected knows, having a sexually transmitted disease is a health problem that causes significant discomfort and embarrassment on its own. On top of this burden, being intimate while carrying an STD, or being intimate with a partner who is dealing with this health problem, puts a strain on the much needed emotional closeness and sexual intercourse necessary to make a baby naturally.

First, let's touch on the latest statistics on the most common sexually transmitted diseases today and how they affect fertility. For the most part, these diseases tend to be bacterial. When a couple is dealing with fertility loss caused by a bacterial infection, fertility returns as soon as the infection is treated and resolved. Please know that being diagnosed with an STD does not mean that you or your partner will inevitably become infertile.

Let's begin with two of the most common sexually transmitted diseases: chlamydia and gonorrhea. These STDs are two of the leading preventable causes of pelvic inflammatory disease (PID) and infertility. If left untreated, about 10 to 15 percent of women with chlamydia will develop PID, according to CDC figures.

Chlamydia can also cause infection of the fallopian tubes without any warning signs. PID and "silent" infection in the upper genital tract may result in permanent damage to the fallopian tubes, uterus, and surrounding tissues, which can lead to fertility problems.

Also according to the CDC:

An estimated 2.86 million cases of chlamydia and 820,000 cases of gonorrhea occur annually in the United States.

Most women infected with chlamydia or gonorrhea have no symptoms.

Do you now understand why it is so important to consider possible undetected, underlying STDs as factors in fertility challenges? What most concerns me is the fact that the majority of women who have either (or both) chlamydia or gonorrhea "have no symptoms."

STDs are not just inconvenient and uncomfortable. They are dangerous. Not just because they cause problems within the reproductive system, but also because they affect our very sexuality and interfere with intimacy. Remember, all must be well in all the vital areas—physical, emotional, mental and sexual—to make a baby.

Although often subtle and overlooked, there are a number of symptoms that mean you may have an STD.

Normally, these symptoms occur around two to three weeks after the initial unprotected sexual contact.

Chlamydia. If left untreated, chlamydia can make it difficult for a woman to get pregnant.

This all too common STD that affects both men and women can cause serious, permanent damage to a woman's reproductive system. This makes it difficult or impossible for her to conceive. And that's not all. If a woman with a chlamydia infection does conceive, she faces great risk for an ectopic pregnancy—that is, a pregnancy that occurs outside the womb—which is potentially fatal.

People who have this very common STD usually have no symptoms. And if there are symptoms they take a while to show up—several weeks after unprotected sex with an infected partner. Sadly, even when there are no symptoms, the damage to the reproductive system has begun from the initial contraction of the infection.

Women with chlamydia may experience: *an abnormal, vaginal discharge.*

Men with chlamydia may: *become sterile; experience pain and swelling in one or both testicles (although this is less common).*

Both men and women with chlamydia may experience: *a thick discharge; a burning, painful sensation when urinating; urethritis (inflammation of the urethra); pelvic pain.*

Men and women are also susceptible to being infected with chlamydia in their rectum. This happens as a result of unprotected anal sex or it can be spread from another infected area of the body, such as the vagina.

Again, these infections often cause no symptoms. If symptoms occur, men and women with chlamydia can experience: *anal, rectal pain; rectal bleeding; anal discharge.*

Gonorrhea. Most women infected with gonorrhea do not have any symptoms whatsoever. When a woman does experience symptoms, they are often so mild she may brush it off as simply being a vaginal or bladder infection. Even though the symptoms are mild or nonexistent, this STD puts women at risk for severe health complications.

If symptoms do show up, women with gonorrhea may experience:

- *an increase in vaginal discharge; usually yellow or cloudy green in color*

- *yeast infection*

- *pain or burning during urination*

- *vaginal spotting and bleeding between menstrual cycles*

- *and, of course, pelvic inflammation*

Again, most men with gonorrhea have no symptoms. If symptoms do show up, men with gonorrhea may experience:

- *burning during urination*
- *a yellow, white, or green discharge from the penis*
- *swollen, inflamed, painful testicles (this symptom happens less often)*

With gonorrhea, just as with chlamydia, rectal infections can also develop in both men and women. These infections may not cause any symptoms. If symptoms do occur, they may include:

- *anal itch*
- *rectal and/or anal soreness*
- *discharge*
- *rectal bleeding*
- *pain during bowel movements*

As stated earlier, chlamydia and gonorrhea are known as precursors to pelvic inflammatory disease (PID), a major cause of infertility in women if left untreated. One in every eight women with a history of PID experiences difficulties conceiving a baby. Besides untreated STDs, other factors associated with developing PID are:

- *having more than one sex partner*
- *having a sex partner who has sex partners other than you*
- *having had PID before*
- *being sexually active and age 25 or younger*
- *regular douching*
- *using an intrauterine device (IUD) for birth control*

Although symptoms are mild and most times women attribute them to other challenges, a woman with PID will notice:

- unexplained fevers
- pain below the belly button in the lower abdomen
- bleeding and/or pain after sexual intercourse
- a burning, painful sensation when urinating
- bleeding between menstrual cycles
- a discharge along with a foul odor from the vagina

Are you or your partner experiencing any of these issues? If so, then consider the reason for your delayed conception may be rooted in PID.

Bacterial vaginosis (BV) is another cause of PID. This bacterial vaginal infection is caused when too much of certain bacteria changes the normal balance of bacteria in the vagina. This is the most common vaginal infection in women ages 15 to 44. Not surprisingly, as with other STDs, most women with BV do not have symptoms. When symptoms do occur, women with BV may experience:

- pain, itching, and a burning sensation in the vagina
- a slight gray or white vaginal discharge
- a fishy, musty, vaginal odor, particularly after sexual intercourse
- pain and burning when urinating
- uncomfortable itching around the outside of the vaginal lips

Human papilloma virus (HPV), also known as venereal warts or genital warts, is the most common sexually transmitted infection (STI). HPV is so prevalent that, according to the CDC, nearly all sexually active men and women will get it at some point in their lives. Research shows there are about one million new cases found every year. This infection affects the uterus, fallopian tubes, ovaries, cervix, and the anal and vaginal areas. How does HPV affect fertility? Most times, infertility results from having this infection. HPV can also increase your risk of developing pre-cancerous or cancerous cells in your cervix, which has a direct affect on your fertility and your pregnancy. Cervical cancer can be treated, also through naturopathic medicine and holistic medicine, if it is caught early.

Yes, I understand, that this is a lot of information to absorb. But know that there is a way to help your body heal from STDs, overcome your challenges, and increase fertility. To give you hope, I will share the story of Sonia.

Sonia came to see me for help with her fertility in December of 2005. She was 39 years old at the time and had a twelve-year-old son, whom she conceived with no problems. Years ago, her relationship with her son's father ended. At this point in her life, she was in a new relationship, and she and her new partner desperately wanted to have a child together.

During her consultation, I learned that Sonia had miscarried a month and a half earlier. Her doctor explained she had a sac that was growing but no fetus, her uterine walls were weak, and so she miscarried. Sonia suffered with PID. Every month for the past few years, she experienced severe pelvic pain. She also shared with me that she had contracted a STD from her ex-husband, which was one of the reasons why she divorced him.

As I usually do with my fertility patients, I explained the process of using the Essential Female Herbal Fertility program. I also recommended two additional herbs. I mentioned one of them earlier: *Pau D'Arco.* The other is known for its potent bacterial and viral fighting properties: *Olive Leaf Extract.* Together, these herbs would help Sonia's body fight off the underlying infection causing her PID, recover from the infection, and promote healing of her uterus and the rest of her reproductive system.

After two full months of following my herbal recommendations, Sonia and her partner again began trying to conceive. Two months was enough time, I felt, for her uterus to become strong and allow her body to recover from the miscarriage as well. Happily, she conceived soon after. On May 22, 2006, Sonia called my office to share the joyous news: she was having another boy!

As far as STDs go, one of the scariest is herpes. Over 80% of Americans with genital herpes (HSV-2) are unaware of their infection. The infection can spread from person to person without producing the feeling of any of the typical symptoms (or any visible symptoms).

There is a definitive test, called the IgG, that looks for antibodies in the blood that would be present to combat the herpes virus. The presence of specific antibodies can tell you which type of herpes you have: HSV1 (oral herpes) or HSV2 (genital herpes).

What is the difference between the two? Genital herpes has way too much stigma attached to it because what shows up on people's lips is actually the same as what shows up on the genitals, though we see its presence on the genitals as more serious. Genital herpes (HSV2) can show up on the mouth, but is much less likely because the HSV2 virus prefers to be in the warm, moist environment of the genitals.

Why is this a fertility concern? Even at birth, babies can pick up the herpes virus going through the birth canal and vagina, which risks blindness, brain damage, and even death for the child.

Use the recommended *Pau D'Arco* and *Olive Leaf Extract* mentioned in this chapter—along with St. John's Wort—for a minimum of three to six months to help the body fight the herpes viruses (and against viruses in general).

Yes, it is possible to have a baby even if your reproductive system and your sex life have suffered from a sexually transmitted disease or infection. I've shared the proof. Rejoice in the possibility of restoring your fertility and delighting in the little miracle to come!

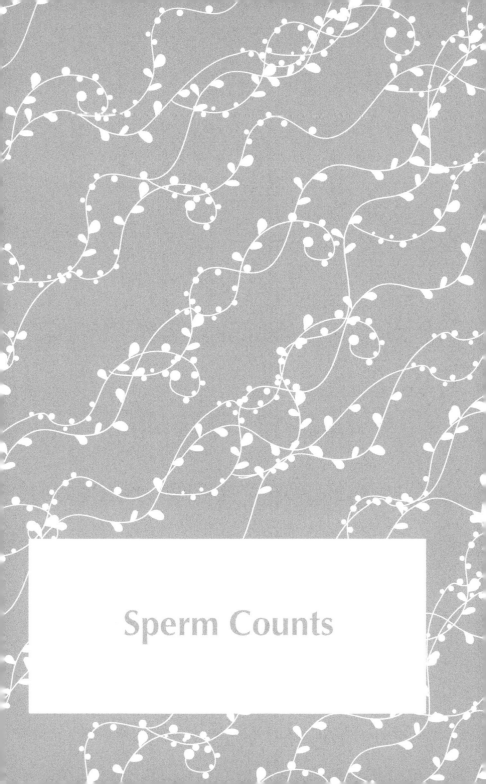

Sperm Counts

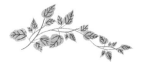

I always tell my fertility patients, it takes two to tango. In other words: it takes both a fertile woman and a fertile man to make a baby happen. His state of health and balance are equally of utmost importance to hers in achieving their dream of becoming parents through a natural pregnancy. Most women feel that they are the ones with the problem and that the man is not the cause of their delayed conception. This is especially true for a woman who hasn't yet had a child, but the man who is her partner has a child or children from a previous relationship. Typically in cases like these, the woman immediately assumes that her man is obviously not the one with the fertility problem because he has impregnated another woman—or multiple women—in the past.

This is so far from the truth. The state of health of a man at the time he fathered that child or children does not necessarily mean his state of health is the same at this very moment. His sperm count, mobility, and motility most definitely could have changed since then. For this reason, it is important to consider a man's health and sperm counts when it comes to fertility.

Among couples with fertility challenges, as most gyne-cologists and obstetricians would agree, the man is just about as likely to be the problem as the woman. Based on numerous medical studies, the man is the cause of the fertility problem about a third of the time. About another third of the time, the woman is the cause of the problem. Sometimes no cause can be found. A study by the World Health Organization (WHO) found that in 20 percent of in-fertility cases the problem was predominantly the male, in 38 percent the problem was predominantly female, in 27 percent abnormalities were found in both partners, and in the remaining 15 percent no clear-cut cause of infertility was identified.

A man is considered infertile if he hasn't been able to get a woman who is healthy and has no reproductive system complications pregnant after at least one year of trying to conceive. Let me explain male fertility in simple terms, al-though it truly is a complex process. How does a man get a woman pregnant? First and foremost, a man must produce healthy sperm. What is healthy sperm? During puberty, the formation of a man's reproductive organs and growth are important.

The testicles, or at least one of a man's testicles, must be functioning properly. To be fertile, a man requires normal spermatogenesis—that is, the development of the sperm cells within the male reproductive organs, the testes. His body must produce healthy levels of testosterone and other hormones must also be in balance to initiate and maintain normal spermatogenesis. Sperm then has to be carried by the semen. When the testicles have produced sperm, the vas deferens—thick-walled tubes in the male reproductive system that transport sperm cells—carry them until they mix with semen to then be ejaculated out of the penis.

The amount of sperm in the semen is crucial. If the number of sperm in the semen (sperm count) is too low, this decreases the chances that one of the sperm will fertilize his partner's egg. And this causes fertility problems.

What is 'normal' sperm count? Normal sperm count is a count within the range of 15 million to 150 million per milliliter of semen. The total ejaculated sperm count should also be between 22 million and 39 million (or more) per ejaculation. A man is diagnosed with low sperm count if he has fewer than 10 million sperm per milliliter of semen or less than 22 million per ejaculated sperm. If a man does not have enough candidates available to fertilize an egg, difficulties getting pregnant arise.

Sperm count is not all a man has to be concerned about. Normal sperm formation and sperm mobility and motility are also factors in having healthy sperm to make baby.

What is normal sperm formation, or morphology? A report by the Mayo Clinic explains, "Normal sperm have oval heads and long tails, which work together to propel them forward. While not as important a factor as sperm quantity or movement, the more sperm you have with a normal shape and structure, the more likely you are to be fertile."

There you have it: blunt and to the point. So, are you a man dealing with sperm count, formation, mobility and motility issues affecting your fertility? Now that you have a firm understanding of the qualities of unhealthy sperm, let's discuss some of the causes.

Factors that contribute to sperm problems and cause male fertility problems in general are:

- *disease of the testes*
- *problems with sperm transportation — that is, the process of how sperm travel from the testes to culminate in ejaculation*
- *problems related to the pituitary and/or hypothalamus glands (these glands are parts of the brain that signal the testes to produce sperm and testosterone)*

Are you a man over 30 years of age having difficulty getting your partner pregnant? The age of a man also plays a significant role in fertility. With age, the proportion of normal sperm and the ability for sperm to have good mobility decreases and affects fertility in a man. According to the U.S. National Library of Medicine, studies have consistently shown that increasing male age is associated with increasing the time it takes to achieve conception and decreasing rates of pregnancy. In one study to determine the effect of age on time needed to achieve pregnancy, researchers assessed surveys from 8,559 couples who had achieved pregnancy. After adjusting for the age of the female partner, conception during a 12-month period was 30 percent less likely for men over age 40 than for men younger than age 30. Similarly, research from the Mayo Clinic shows that it takes longer for men in their mid-30s and early 40s to achieve pregnancy with their partner than it does for younger men.

For any man with low sperm count, poor sperm formation, and/ or low sperm mobility and motility, regardless of his age, know that there is a solution. There is hope for making a baby, naturally. Consider the story of my fertility patients, Ella and Jose.

Ella came to see me in early 2010. She explained that she and Jose, both in their twenties at the time, had been together for three years. Although they had decided to have a baby together after celebrating one year as a couple, and had been having unprotected sex regularly for two years, she still had not conceived. Ella was concerned she was the cause of their fertility problem. Yet, after consulting her conventional doctor and having numerous tests done, she was told she was healthy and should have no problems conceiving.

She further explained that she had to push Jose to go to his doctor to get his own tests done to determine why they still were not getting pregnant after trying for so long. Jose was told by his doctor he had low sperm count. He was producing only about 10 million sperm per milliliter; in addition, his sperm mobility and motility were low. As Ella continued to tell me their story, she began to get upset and paused for a moment. She hesitated but finally confided in me that she felt the cause of Jose's fertility problem was the fact that he smoked marijuana (cannabis) and had been doing so from the time he was a young teenager.

Could marijuana be one of the causes of Jose's fertility problems? To quote a study published by the U.S. National Library of Medicine: "reports (show) that acute cannabinoid treatments affects the quality and quantity of spermatozoa produced by the testis." I shared Ella's feeling about Jose's marijuana habit. I first told Ella that there are a number of causes for sperm problems in men. One of those causes, which I touched on earlier, is possible problems of the pituitary and/or hypothalamus glands in the brain.

Marijuana affects a variety of hormones that are regulated by the hypothalamus. We know that hormonal balance is extremely important to fertility. Hormones secreted by the pituitary gland are of major importance to reproduction in the male.

Marijuana affects this gland as well. It is an important fact for men to know, especially any men who enjoy "getting stoned" and believe smoking marijuana is harmless. In a major study conducted on laboratory animals such as rats, mice, and monkeys, chronic exposure to marijuana and the various cannabinoids it contains was shown to affect the function of several reproductive organs.

Yes. The fact that Jose smoked marijuana was most surely a factor to be considered as a cause of his infertility.

Now, back to Ella and Jose's story... When Ella was done pouring out her heart, sharing her distress about Jose's habit and her desire to have a baby, I began to speak compassionately and comfort her.

I let Ella know that I would do everything in my power to help her and Jose fulfill their dream of having a baby together. If Jose was willing to work with Ella and follow my recommendations, then we would be able to overcome his fertility problem.

As I stressed to Ella, it was imperative that she begin her Essential Female Herbal Fertility Program that very day, although she was told she was healthy and my tests confirmed the same.

It will always help to increase fertility wherever we can. I also suggested that she and Jose come back to my office together the next week.

That way, I could devote the time to talk to Jose and ensure he understood exactly what he needed to do as far as lifestyle changes, as well as the herbs he needed to use, to dramatically increase—indeed, just about double—his sperm count in one to two months and also to increase his sperm mobility and motility.

True to their commitment, both Ella and Jose accepted my recommendations and began their respective programs. To increase his fertility, Jose made some "sacrifices" as he put it, and stopped smoking marijuana. In addition, he began his Essential Male Herbal Fertility Program.

In that program, I have already included herbs and a potent mineral, *Zinc*, which is known to double sperm count in about thirty to forty-five days when taken in high dosages (I will share more details and specific dosage guideline in the glossary).

Additionally, to increase his chances of impregnating Ella by 21 percent by increasing sperm mobility and motility, I added the following supplement to his essential program: *Vitamin E with Selenium.*

A little over two-and-a-half months later, Ella called my office to share the good news. She and Jose were pregnant! They are now the happy parents of an energetic, lively little boy who loves to run.

Many of you may be able to relate to Ella and Jose's story, or know a couple struggling to conceive who may be dealing with similar sperm-related challenges. Men, I've shared what you need to do to make a baby a reality. Now, it's your choice to do what must be done to achieve that dream.

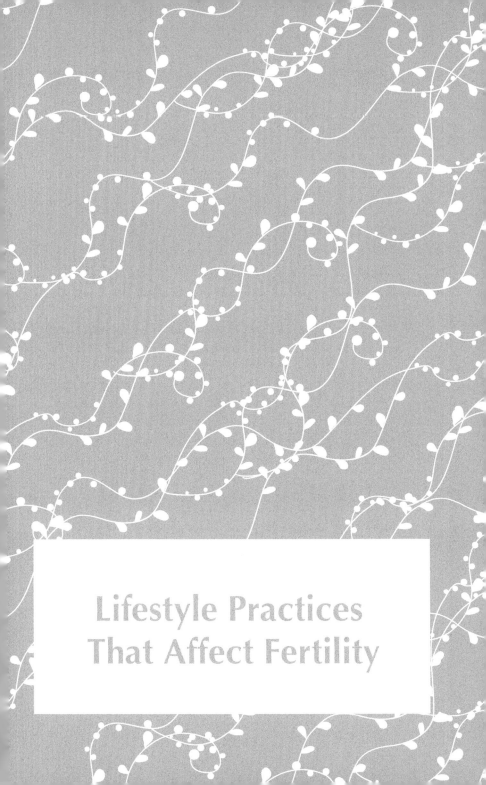

Lifestyle Practices
That Affect Fertility

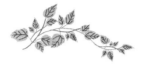

If you knew you were doing something every day that was interfering with your fertility, you would just stop doing it, wouldn't you? Many couples simply aren't aware of how their everyday habits, and even their surroundings, are holding them back from having that adoring baby they've been dreaming about. It would feel great to know that all your daily habits and routine activities are helping to ensure the conception of a baby, wouldn't it? Can you think of some habits that you and/or your partner have developed, or some activities that you and/or partner frequently carry out, that could be hindering your fertility?

Let's start with smoking. We have already touched upon how smoking marijuana can hinder your chances of conceiving. According to research cited in *Science* magazine, marijuana use at even "moderate" levels was found to stop ovulation in monkeys for 103 to 135 days. Research further indicated that the THC in marijuana may be directly toxic to the developing egg. With marijuana use, neural pathways into the hypothalamus, a gland that regulates the reproductive cycle, are being suppressed. Clearly, women who are attempting to get pregnant, as well as women who are pregnant, should not smoke marijuana.

Then, there's that nasty nicotine habit. Yes, smoking cigarettes (or cigars) can impair fertility in both women and men. In women, as extensive research shows, smoking affects how receptive the uterus is to the egg. And in men, smoking can reduce sperm production and damage DNA.

Need more reasons to kick the habit? Consider the following research findings:

According to researchers at Johns Hopkins, couples in which both spouses smoked had a 28 percent decrease in fertility.

According to research in The American Journal of Epidemiology, male smokers show an increase in sperm abnormalities.

According to the Journal of the American Medical Association(JAMA), female smokers face higher infertility. In a large national study, women who smoked were three to four times more likely than nonsmokers to have taken longer than a year to conceive.

The good news? Research also indicates that smoking's toxic effect on fertility is temporary.

According to the Fertility Sterility Journal, sperm counts in male smokers are, on average, 13 to 17 percent lower than nonsmokers.

However, any reduction in sperm count caused by smoking is reversible. A study of smokers who were followed for up to fifteen months after stopping smoking reported remarkable rebounds in former smokers' sperm counts, increases between 50 and 800 percent.

A study published in Obstetrics & Gynecology investigated the effects of cigarette smoking, past and present, in 499 women regarding their fertility and ovarian function. The characteristics of ovarian function were compared among current smokers, past smokers, and nonsmokers. The conclusion?

Cigarette smoking is definitely associated with a prolonged, adverse effect on ovarian function. Compared with nonsmokers, current smokers had a dramatically reduced pregnancy rate. However, the differences between the fertility rates of nonsmokers and past smokers were not statistically significant.

If you or your partner is hooked on this deadly habit and you want to get pregnant, stop smoking. Also, avoid exposure to secondary smoke.

And what about a couple who uses illegal substances such as cocaine? I would imagine you and your partner not only want to focus on eliminating those lifestyle practices that impede conception but also want to give birth to a healthy baby. Cocaine use in men before conceiving has been linked to abnormal development in offspring according to a study cited in *The Journal of the American Medical Association*, (JAMA).

The suspected cause is that cocaine binds onto the sperm and thus finds its way into the egg at fertilization.

Along with secondary smoke, there is a long, long list of environmental toxins that are hazardous to fertility in both men and women. Here are some findings you should heed:

Working with pesticides, many of which cause infertility in men. According to a study in the American Journal of Industrial Medicine, men experiencing infertility were found to be employed in agricultural/pesticide related jobs ten times more often than men with no fertility challenges.

Wearing briefs or boxers washed with standard laundry detergent may lower sperm count. In a study reported in Epidemiology, men with higher than average urine levels of nonylphenol, a chemical agent commonly used in commercial laundry detergents, were up to 21 times more likely to have low sperm counts than men with lower than average urine levels of this chemical.

Autoantibodies. These are "renegade" immune system components which mistakenly attack the person's own body. When the immune cells attack either the sperm or egg, this definitely impacts fertility. In a study published in the Fertility Sterility Journal, the rate of autoimmune antibodies was 33 percent in women unable to deliver a baby to full term and 0 percent in a control group of women with successful pregnancies. (Research shows that autoantibodies are higher in people exposed to certain pesticides.)

Breathing in car exhaust can decrease fertility in women. As a study in Environmental Health Perspectives (EHP) found, exposure to a common car exhaust compound caused a significant reduction in fertility in test animals, particularly affecting the ovaries.

Exposure to chlordane, a pesticide most commonly used to control termites. Research suggests that chlordane exposure leads to lower sperm counts and damage to the sperm and testicles. Based on expert estimates, approximately 75 percent of U.S. homes contain breathable chlordane.

Surprised? Well, that's far from all. Your sofa, carpet and even bedroom furniture may be affecting your ability to conceive a baby. A study, also in EHP, showed a link between exposure to flame retardant chemicals and fertility challenges in women. Flame retardant chemicals, called PBDEs, are added to foam rubber in couch cushions, carpet pads, and bedding materials. Women with 8 to 10 times higher levels of PBDEs in their blood than women with no exposure were 30 percent less likely to become pregnant. The European Union banned PBDEs in 2002, but a ban has not been enacted in the U.S. Not surprisingly, Americans have 20 times more PBDEs in their blood than Europeans.

Another everyday household hazard to fertility is a chemical substance widely found in plastic wrap, vinyl shower curtains, and carpet padding, as well as some air fresheners, perfumes, colognes, shampoos, and body creams. Used to soften plastics and smooth the texture of other products, it is called phthalates. In one study, couples unable to conceive were found to have three to five times higher urine levels of phthalates than couples who had achieved pregnancy.

These chemicals mimic natural hormones needed for conception and may be interfering with this process. Phthalates are still allowed in the U.S. but have been banned in the European Union.

As you see, environmental toxins play a huge role in fertility problems. I understand this is a lot to take in. But wouldn't you rather know all this than be in the dark? Isn't having that baby, the family you dream of, this important?

Let's continue with the discussion. Gentlemen, are you drinking, bathing, and showering in the right kind of water? Once again, EHP linked a decrease in sperm quality to a chemical: chlorine in water. Men exposed to chlorinated water (whether through drinking, bathing, showering, or even swimming) were found to have reduced sperm motility and a lower sperm count. How would you reduce this exposure? Drink pure clean filtered water. In *The Lancet*, a report showed the link between male infertility and chemicals in drinking water. Drinking water from the Thames Water Supply in the United Kingdom was pinpointed as the cause of lower sperm counts and increases in abnormally shaped sperm. Also, buy a chlorine shower filter to remove this chemical from the water entering your home.

Are you or your partner a dentist or a dental assistant? Sadly, this may also be a factor hindering your possibilities of conception. Dental workers are exposed to higher than normal rates of mercury, adhesives and chemicals used in plastics. And, based on a recent study, they have a higher rate of pregnancy problems. In a sample of dental workers, spontaneous abortions, stillbirths, and congenital defects occurred at a rate of 24 percent compared to 11 percent for the control group. Five out of six malformations were spina bifida.

Are you a fireman? *Harvard Health Letter* shared the following finding: Firemen appear to produce an unusually high number of abnormal sperm and be less fertile than other males. The likely cause is exposure to toxic smoke emitted when carpets, furniture and paints—which are typically made from synthetic or plastic-based compounds—catch on fire. Burning plastic at low temperatures creates high levels of the highly toxic compound dioxin.

Yes, your choice of occupation or profession can impact fertility. The Organization for Economic Cooperation and Development (OECD) and the European Economic Community (EEC) did the following study regarding the risk of miscarriage associated with exposure to chemicals in the workplace. The findings are alarming:

- *perchlorethylene (dry cleaning)........4.7 times greater risk*
- *trichloroethylene (dry cleaning)......3.1 times greater risk*
- *paint thinners ....2.1 times greater risk*
- *paint strippers .... 2.1 times greater risk*
- *glycol ethers (found in paints)............ 2.9 times greater risk*

And if there is a risk of miscarriage, it is important to understand there is also a risk of delayed conception. Even with all this overwhelming information, in truth, very little is known about the reproductive dangers of many chemicals. Studies have found increased risk of fertility problems in both women and men linked to exposure to textile dyes, dry cleaning chemicals, anti-rust agents, welding, plastic manufacturing, and simply handling antibiotics. My advice for all couples trying to conceive a child is to limit, if not avoid, exposure to chemical substances as much as possible. Read labels. Purchase products made from all-natural materials. Also, if possible, avoid being exposed to high amounts of pollutants and smog.

Now, what about alcohol? Are you a couple who enjoys a glass of wine with dinner every night? If so, that habit could be contributing to challenges with getting pregnant. Many studies have found that regular drinkers have decreased fecundability—that is, the probability of achieving pregnancy the natural way. A study in *Science News* demonstrated just how dramatically alcohol reduces fertilization success. In experiments with test animals given "intoxicating" doses of alcohol 24 hours prior to mating, the rate of conception was reduced by 50 percent.

What about that morning coffee habit? Remember, I mentioned toxic caffeine as a cause of fertility problems in chapter 2. Here is more research to support this connection:

One study, reported in the American Journal of Epidemiology, found a 50 percent reduction in fertility for women who drank more than one cup of coffee per day and an 80 percent increased risk in failure to conceive within one year among women who drank more four or more cups of coffee per day.

Another study, of 1,909 women in Connecticut, found the risk of not conceiving for 12 months (the usual definition of infertility) was 55 percent higher for women drinking one cup of coffee per day, 100 percent higher for women drinking one-and-one-half to three cups of coffee per day, and 176 percent higher for women drinking more than three cups of coffee per day.

Research in JAMA revealed how coffee increases miscarriage risk. Coffee drinking before and during pregnancy was associated with over twice the risk of miscarriage when the mother consumed two to three cups of coffee per day.

Ladies, if having a baby is what you most desire, discontinue drinking coffee altogether.

And what about men who drink coffee? Are you one that does intake this beverage and has had problems getting your partner pregnant? Another report in the same

American Journal of Epidemiology found a negative effect of male caffeine intake for those who drank more than 700 milligrams of caffeine per day. Don't think about measuring the milligrams of coffee in your mug! Stop drinking coffee altogether to increase your chances of conception.

So, are you willing to make some changes now that all this has been made clear? Let's discuss how to overcome all this toxic exposure. Understand and have hope, my friends, that following my recommended Essential Herbal Fertility Programs will help to protect against our toxic world, cleanse and purify the blood, and strengthen the reproductive system respectively in a man and a woman to increase your ability to conceive.

With that comfort in mind, what are other practices you can start doing today to help your fertility?

First, reduce stress. Stress is linked to abnormal sperm production. One way to both relax is to go take frequent walks together, holding hands, go to spas together and get side-by-side massages! One factor I have noticed is that although a couple may be on the same page about wanting to have a child together, they may not see eye to eye with many other factors, and this causes undue stress between the two.

While getting a couples' massage, try holding hands as the soft music carries you both away. Concentrate on the nurturing you are both receiving and deserve. Melt as one under the hands of your massage therapists. It's a simple formula: decrease stress, increase your fertility.

And get more sleep. Turn off that late night show and allow your bodies to rest! Studies show 25 percent of American couples have fertility problems because they are just too fatigued, too tired to make love! Bluntly put: how can making a baby come easy if you and your partner hardly have sex? And believe it or not, gentlemen, even too much sex is not healthy. Other research shows that sex on a constant basis—more than three times per week—tends to reduce sperm quality. I recommend affectionate gestures always be practiced. This maintains a beautiful bond between the two of you that carries on to the days you are intimate during her ovulation cycle so that conceiving a baby is joyous, loving and sensual.

On a related note... Men: avoid overheating your scrotum and testicles! According to World Health Organization (WHO) researchers, the ideal temperature for sperm production is three to four degrees below normal body temperature. Any warmer will affect sperm count, slashing it by about 40 percent per one-degree rise. Temporary overheating of the testicles can result from exposure to things such as saunas, hot tubs, heating blankets, or even waterbeds. Other research has shown that men who sleep in waterbeds are up to four times more likely to suffer fertility problems than those who prefer a traditional mattress.

Frequent bike riding and wearing tight clothing can temporarily trap heat in those vital private parts as well, although tight underwear has not been shown scientifically to cause any increase in testicular heat. Nevertheless, a change to looser clothing couldn't hurt when fertility is a concern.

Other factors that can cause overheating and decreased sperm production inside the testicles include climate and work environment. According to one study, semen specimens obtained in New Orleans during the summer had significantly lower sperm concentration than samples provided at other times of year. These findings suggest that men may be more fertile in cooler climates and during cooler months of the year. Sperm counts are about 30 percent lower in summer. While heat may play a role, the seasonal rise and fall may be a legacy of our ancestors who bred seasonally.

In addition, exposure to heat over an extended period of time, such as in occupations which involve long hours of sitting, may result in impaired fertility. One experiment showed that scrotal temperature rises by up to 2.2 degrees within two hours of driving a vehicle, putting truckers and taxi drivers at risk for a low sperm count.

As for those who work with computers, another recent study warned young men to limit the time they use laptops on their laps after tests showed the heat from the battery might impair sperm production. Research also indicates that men who balance their laptops on their laps risk infertility problems because of the combination of pressing their legs together, which constricts the scrotum, and the heat from the laptop, which raises its temperature. One study found that after sitting with a computer in their laps for 15 minutes, men's scrotal temperatures had risen 1.8 degrees, and 2.8 degrees after an hour. It is not known whether the effects of the exposure would cause permanent damage, but the study recommended that men keep laptops off their laps to avoid the potential for "irreversible changes."

As far as damage from other factors, such as saunas, hot tubs, and heating blankets, it is believed that sperm generally recover quickly from heat exposure, so a man's sperm count should return to normal within about a week. However, at least one study has shown that the production of sperm is a process requiring approximately three months, which suggests that even when a factor that may be harmful to production is taken away, a normal sperm count may not occur again for at least three months.

In addition to reducing stress, sleeping more, and keeping cool, get more healthy exposure to natural sunlight. Researchers have discovered that Vitamin D plays a significant role in reproductive physiology. To avoid Vitamin D deficiency, what do I recommend? That men, and it won't hurt if women do the same, spend at least 15 minutes every day, preferably in the morning, sunbathing in the nude or allowing the sun's rays to caress your face. The best way for us to absorb Vitamin D is by exposing ourselves to the sun for this short amount of time and by this practice increase fertility.

Ladies, to increase your chances of fertility, continue with practices that help to reduce stress in your lives. I frequently recommend that my patients begin practicing mild yoga and deep breathing, and encourage continuing those practices during the pregnancy as well. Personally, I began my yoga practice during my pregnancy; even at eight months, I was doing triangle headstands. I feel yoga tones the reproductive system, making the uterus a strong 'home' for baby to develop, and also decreases labor pains, length of labor, and complications. Why do I feel this is so? Because I had a natural birth 16 years ago, and gave birth to my son in 48 minutes.

Next, I recommend that couples use only natural sexual lubricants during intercourse, if needed. Studies have shown that chemical sexual lubricants affect fertility. In one recent study conducted by researchers at the State University of New York Upstate Medical Center in Syracuse, semen samples were collected from 22 healthy donors in a test tube. Four types of sexual lubricants were added from store shelves. What were the findings? All of the four sexual lubricants impaired sperms' motility. To achieve conception, it is necessary that the sperm have the ability to move and to move forward.

Sperm must make its way through the vagina, uterus, and fallopian tubes in a swift manner in order to successfully fertilize an egg.

And lastly, exercise. I can't stress enough how vitally important it is for both the man and woman to exercise to increase the likelihood of conception. Exercise helps balance hormones and increase circulation throughout the body, all factors, as you have learned, that support fertility. However, both should practice mild exercise because strenuous exercise that is too intense can actually hinder fertility. Exercising together is another way to increase the loving bond between the two of you, and also has been shown to increase sexual desire (libido) in both!

So there you have it. Everyday habits matter! Start today to make the required positive changes to improve your fertility, and you will be well on your way to becoming parents who will rejoice in a little creation, a tiny miracle of your very own.

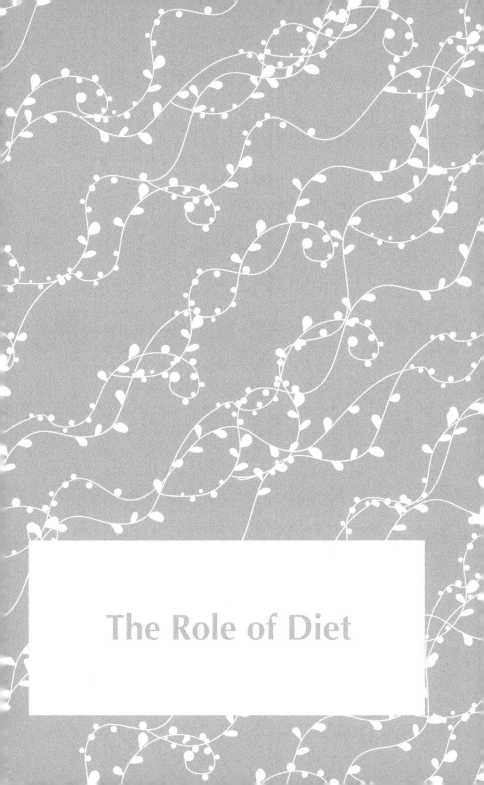

The Role of Diet

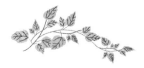

What we eat affects our overall health. Fertility is another factor very much affected by how we nourish our bodies. Diet is of utmost importance. It is difficult for the body to allow conception without good, proper, healthy nutrition. Before even trying to conceive a baby together, both partners should be balanced and as healthy as possible to ensure the proper development of their baby-to-be.

So, what specific foods harm or weaken the reproductive system of a man and a woman, respectively? In the previous chapter, I alerted you to the fertility hazards of drinking coffee. Let's discuss foods a couple should stop eating—as well as foods a couple should start eating or eat more of—to increase their chances of conception.

Now, doesn't it seem like the healthier and more organic we eat, the better? Men, in your case, research from *The Lancet shows* men who eat mostly organic foods produce a whopping 43 percent more sperm than those men who don't. Fertility rates were significantly decreased for couples with higher levels of male exposure to pesticides, a common ingredient in commercially grown and manufactured food.

Gentlemen, emphasize organic foods. Your body, your partner, and your future baby are worth it. Especially, eat organic tomatoes, which are rich in lycopene. According to studies on the effects of lycopene and fertility in men, reported in the *Asian Journal of Andrology* and cited in the U.S. National Library of Medicine, lycopene is a possible treatment option for male fertility problems because of its potent antioxidant properties. Oxidative stress, essentially an imbalance between the production of free radicals and the body's ability to counteract their harmful effects, has been linked to decreased sperm count, viability, and motility.

By neutralizing free radicals, lycopene could reduce the incidence of oxidative stress and make sperm less vulnerable to damage. Studies of the use of lycopene supplements have shown promising results in increasing sperm count and viability, which increase the chances of normal sperm fertilizing an egg. In clinical trials of men with fertility challenges, taking 4 to 8 milligrams of lycopene daily for three to twelve months was related to an increase in pregnancy rates.

Men, your body is your temple. If you have not been treating that temple with care by eating healthy, organic foods, and you are having problems conceiving, I strongly recommend taking a *Lycopene* supplement in addition to the Essential Male Fertility Herbal Program.

Need more reasons to eat organic? Do you know the harmful effects of genetically modified organism (GMO) foods? First, for those of you who aren't quite sure what kind of food that is, a GMO is a plant developed through a process in which a copy of a desired gene or section of genetic material from one plant or organism is placed in another plant.

There are nine GMO commercial crops available in the U.S.: soybeans, corn, potato, papaya, alfalfa, sugar beets, cotton, canola, and summer squash. While many debate the safety of GMOs, a study by the American Academy of Environmental Medicine (AAEM) concluded: "There is more than a casual association between GMO foods and adverse health effects." The Austrian Health Ministers reported that fertility rates, as well as immune system health, suffered dramatically due to GMO exposure. Based on their research, people who regularly consumed GMO foods were more likely to fall ill, age faster, and have a more difficult time conceiving and staying pregnant.

This goes along with reducing foods laced with pesticides and other chemicals. What is the better choice? Eat organic foods. It bears repeating: your body, your partner, and your future baby are worth the extra effort and investment.

How many of you men out there like to eat big beefy burgers and thick juicy steaks? The average American consumes 75 pounds of red meat a year, based on recent USDA figures, and, as surveys show, men tend to eat more red meat than women. Did you know consuming red meat can hinder your chances of becoming a father? In an international study published in the medical journal *Fertility and Sterility*, researchers from Harvard Medical School and Massachusetts General Hospital in the U.S. and Huazhong University of Science and Technology in China analyzed the diets and fertility of 141 men.

Sperm samples from men who ate a diet high in processed meat had less success fertilizing eggs. That should be enough to kill your appetite for burgers and steaks, yes? Red meats are also known to contain harmful amounts of synthetic hormones. Eliminating this from your diet, gentlemen, not only will increase your chances of fertility, but also most definitely make you healthier overall. And I am sure you not only want to help your partner make a baby, but also want to be a healthy, active father who will be around, with vigor and vitality, to watch your child grow.

And what about sugar? As you know, too much sugar is bad for your teeth and your waistline. But what about your sperm? Researchers at the University of Rochester conducted a study of the relationship between consumption of sugar-sweetened beverages and semen quality in healthy young men. Men in the highest quartile of sugary soft drink intake had the lowest percentage of sperm motility. For the sake of your fertility, switch from your preferred sugar-sweetened beverage to refreshing, filtered water.

Think junk foods and fatty foods could be a cause of your fertility challenges? Then you're right. The journal *Human Reproduction* published a study examining the connection between dietary fats and semen quality. Men in the highest third of total fat intake had 43 percent lower total sperm count and 38 percent lower sperm concentration than men in the lowest third. This association was driven by intake of saturated fats. Levels of saturated fatty acids in sperm were also negatively related to sperm concentration, but saturated fat intake was unrelated to sperm levels.

Which 'healthy fat' showed a big difference and promoted healthy sperm in these men? Essential fatty acids (EFAs). Higher intake of omega-3 polyunsaturated fats was related to a more favorable sperm morphology— that is, the percentage of sperm that appear normal when semen is viewed under a microscope. Normal sperm have an oval head with a long tail. Abnormal sperm have head and tail defects such as a large or misshapen head or a crooked or double tail. Men in the highest third of consumption of omega-3 fatty acids had nearly a 2 percent higher normal morphology than men in the lowest third. My recommendation? Add a natural *Omega-3* supplement to your Essential Male Fertility Herbal Program if you are concerned about your sperm concentration.

As too many people know from experience, our unhealthy eating habits have led to an obesity epidemic. What if you are an overweight or obese woman? Could your weight problem be preventing you and your partner from becoming parents? Yes, a high body mass index (BMI) most definitely decreases fertility, especially when it's combined with a sedentary lifestyle. The good news? For women who commit to eating healthier and exercising, gains in fertility can quickly follow. Consider the results of a study in the *New England Journal of Medicine*, involving 574 women with fertility challenges who were either overweight or obese.

Researchers recommended a six-month intervention: a reduction of daily calorie intake to lower BMI by greater than five percent and an increase in physical activity of ten thousand steps daily, plus 30 minutes of moderate exercise two to three times weekly. That regimen would then be followed by infertility treatment. After six months, the women reported weight loss in the range of roughly three to ten pounds. Did any of these "infertile" women conceive? Yes. Twenty-six percent of women in the intervention group achieved natural conception. As this study shows, achieving an optimal BMI increases the chances of achieving natural conception.

So, for young women with a high BMI who are having difficulty getting pregnant, modest weight loss and moderate exercise should be encouraged. Making these lifestyle changes is a much healthier and far less stressful and less costly alternative to conventional infertility treatments.

Excessive weight can also prevent men from fathering a child. Several studies have indicated that obesity has a negative impact on sperm quality. Over the past 30 years, obesity in reproductive-age men has nearly tripled and coincides with an increase in male infertility worldwide. According to an article published in the journal *Spermatogenesis* in the U.S. National Library of Medicine, there is emerging evidence that obesity hinders a man's reproductive potential by not only reducing sperm quality, but also altering the physical and molecular structure of cells in the testes.

Research also shows that the father's obesity at the time of conception impairs embryo health, therefore reducing live birth rates. Obese men are more likely to suffer from elevated blood sugar and blood pressure levels, which have been widely associated with decreased sperm quantity and quality. Losing weight improves not only a man's fertility but also his metabolism and overall health, which directly affects the health of his child.

What should a couple do if both partners are dealing with weight gain or obesity? To start, eat less fatty and junk food and make a commitment to physical activity. You might begin by taking a walk together after dinner. Be comforted: I have taken a sluggish metabolism into account in each respective Essential Fertility Herbal Program, and I have added an herb that begins to stimulate metabolism: *Kelp.*

Now, you know which foods you shouldn't eat and why you shouldn't overeat. So, what should you be eating to increase fertility? I recommend eating much more organic food, particularly all kinds of vegetables, fresh fruit (but no more than one piece per day to prevent excessive, although natural, sugar intake), whole grains, and sea vegetables rich in iodine. If you are not a vegetarian, you can also increase your consumption of seafood— but only well cooked. That means no raw fish, including sushi and ceviche.

For men, focus on foods rich in *Zinc*. Here is a list to help you begin preparing your bodies to conceive:

- *Oysters (not raw)*
- *Crab, Alaska king*
- *Breakfast cereal: fortified with 25 percent of the daily recommended value for zinc (Again, I urge you to buy organic cereals to reduce the intake of processed foods)*
- *Lobster*
- *Baked beans*
- *Chicken: roasted or baked, skin removed, organic*
- *Yogurt: fruit, low-fat (best if organic)*
- *Cashews, dry roasted, organic*
- *Chickpeas*
- • *Swiss cheese (Caution: non-organic dairy has so many synthetic hormones)*
- *Oatmeal*
- *Almonds: dry roasted, organic*

- *kidney beans, cooked*
- *Cheese: cheddar or mozzarella, organic*
- *Peas: green, frozen, cooked, organic*
- *Flounder or sole, cooked*

Another wonderful, soothing food—actually, drink—I recommend that both women and men include in their daily fertility-enhancing diet is green tea. According to a study published in the *American Journal of Public Health*, regularly drinking *Green Tea*, even as little as one cup a day, can double your chances of conceiving a baby. In the study, other caffeinated drinks did not produce the same wonderful effect. (Remember, the caffeine from coffee and even the toxicity of decaffeinated coffee are not recommended.)

Green tea is naturally low in caffeine and has other beneficial properties.) So drink your tea with joy! I recommend at least two cups per day to have an impact on the reproductive system.

What if you and your partner have been practicing bad eating habits for years and years? Take heart. The fertility damage of a poor diet can be reversed. In my Essential Fertility Herbal Programs for both women and men, you will find an herb with amazing nutritional potency: *Alfalfa*. A father herb, alfalfa grows from roots deepest into the ground and is rich in nutrients.

Along with your respective Essential Fertility Herbal Program, make the necessary changes to begin a healthy diet at least three to six months before you begin to act on your desire to conceive. By eating healthy, you will gain physical energy and mental clarity. You will feel better and enjoy sex more, too. Why not start today?

It has been such a blessing in my 20-plus years in practice to have helped so many happy couples with their fertility and to have celebrated the birth of so many healthy babies! I am forever grateful that they have all been successful, joyful pregnancies. Allow me the honor of helping you have the same.

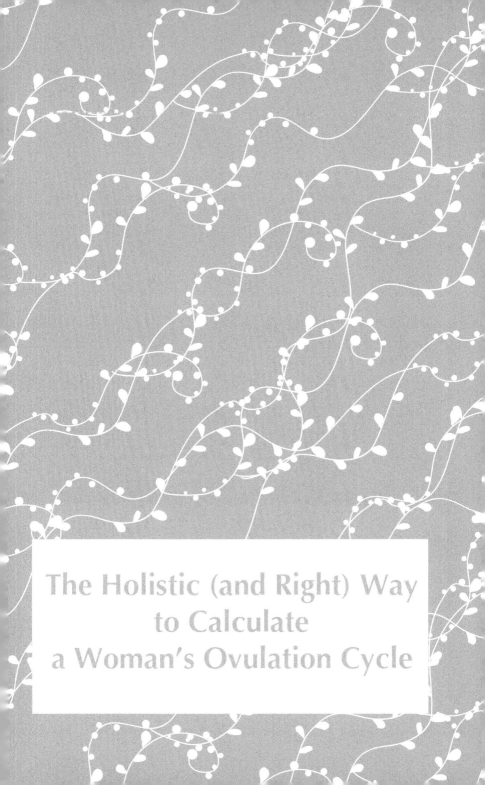

The Holistic (and Right) Way to Calculate a Woman's Ovulation Cycle

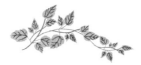

As I discuss the following details about a woman's and a man's body from a holistic and Chinese medicine point of view, I ask that you try to 'unlearn' what you have learned from conventional, allopathic medicine. Imagine a blank slate cleared away of clutter, frustrating information, tips and tricks that you've picked up along the way and that haven't worked for you.

Let's begin with ovulation. Ovulation occurs when a woman's mature egg is released from one of her ovaries, travels down the fallopian tube, and is ready to be fertilized. Nature has shown us every month an egg will mature within one of a woman's ovaries. That is why it is imperative to take advantage of this golden time to conceive a baby.

Each month, a woman ovulates only once: one day during the month. And in truth, we can only guess which day that will be. Every woman's menstrual cycle is unique and not every woman's menstrual cycle is like clockwork. That makes it difficult for any woman to say, "Honey, this day and at this time, we should make that baby!" So, let's look at how I explain to my patients a natural, holistic way of calculating a woman's ovulation cycle.

First, ladies, understand it doesn't matter if you have a twenty-five day menstrual cycle or a twenty-eight day menstrual cycle. Regardless, you are going to begin your countdown the first day of your period.

Now, let me back up just a moment. There are some tools I recommend that you, as a couple, have on hand to calculate what I am about to teach you. First and foremost, you need to obtain a personal diary with a calendar and a writing utensil. In this day and age, I understand there are all kinds of apps and that we all use our cell phones, the one device that can carry and manage pretty much all the information we need for our active lives. But I believe that when we write something down on paper, we better comprehend and remember the given task.

That said, the following is the correct way to take advantage of a woman's ovulation cycle:

JANUARY

SUNDAY	MONDAY	TUESDAY	WEDNESDAY	THURSDAY	FRIDAY	SATURDAY
					1	2
Day 1 3	4	5	6	7	8	9
10	11	12	13	14	15	16
17	18	19	20	21	22	23
24 / 31	25	26	27	28	29	30

Begin counting from the first day of your menstrual period. That is, the first day you see menstrual blood flow, whether it be in the morning or the evening. Write this down on your calendar as Day 1. For example, if you start your period on the third day of the first month of the year, then January 3rd would by Day 1.

Starting with Day 1, count the days, writing in the number of each day on the calendar as you go, until you get to Day 10. Using the same example, Day 10 would be January 12th.

JANUARY

SUNDAY	MONDAY	TUESDAY	WEDNESDAY	THURSDAY	FRIDAY	SATURDAY
					1	2
Day 1 3	Day 2 4	Day 3 5	Day 4 6	Day 5 7	Day 6 8	Day 7 9
Day 8 10	Day 9 11	Day 10 12	13	14	15	16
17	18	19	20	21	22	23
24 / 31	25	26	27	28	29	30

Between day 10 and day 18 is a woman's most fertile time: her ovulation cycle. Now, fill in and start circling days 10, 11, 12... all the way until you arrive at day 18 and stop. These days are the 9 days every month a woman is her most fertile. Continuing with the same exact, you would be most fertile between January 12th and January 20th.

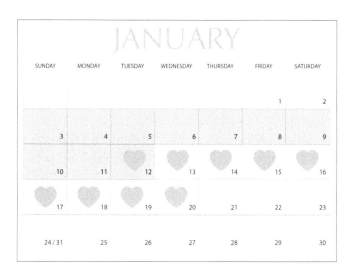

JANUARY

SUNDAY	MONDAY	TUESDAY	WEDNESDAY	THURSDAY	FRIDAY	SATURDAY
					1	2
3	4	5	6	7	8	9
10	11	12	13	14	15	16
17	18	19	20	21	22	23
24 / 31	25	26	27	28	29	30

Here's the catch: a woman ovulates only 1 day out of these 9 days. And we don't know exactly what day that is. So, this is what I recommend to my patients. Once a couple has been balancing their bodies and minds, using their respective Essential Herbal Fertility Program, and has given themselves time, at least 30 to 60 days, to become more fertile, I recommend a 9-day commitment to intimacy when the woman is most fertile. Yes, you and your partner should have sexual intercourse every day for 9 days straight.

I had a husband once label this humorously as the "baby-making-marathon." Do not worry. You will both absolutely want to be intimate as often as possible, given I have included *Damiana* in your respective herbal therapy programs. This herb is known as a wonderfully potent natural aphrodisiac that increases libido, sexual desire and fortifies the male and female reproductive systems!

Let us now discuss sex. Sex should be thought of as a beautiful, exquisite, natural function; Chinese medicine labels it "as natural as clouds and rain." So, what positions increase your likelihood of conception? Let's be blunt: this is just as important as having intercourse the right time of the month to become pregnant.

Now, I am sure we have all heard before that the 'missionary position' is the best position to conceive a baby. Well, in my opinion, this is most definitely one of them. It has been noted that lying down after sex allows the sperm to get to the egg much sooner. The same is believed of lying down during sex.

When a woman is lying horizontally, it allows for a better chance of conception. Let us consider using gravity to your advantage, shall we? Intercourse from behind is another position said to help with conception. But after her partner has ejaculated, the woman should lay relaxed horizontally.

Yes, you can become pregnant by having intercourse in other positions. However, if you both desire to try other positions as you are joyfully enjoying each other, I strongly urge that the man ejaculate while in the missionary position to increase your chances of becoming pregnant.

Chinese medicine emphasizes the preciousness of sex between loving partners. According to the ancient medical text, ***Prescriptions of Life Preservation,*** there are 10 important principles of sex. I believe that these revered principles directly relate to fertility.

1. Preservation of kidney qi (chi), or kidney energy.
Remember how I emphasized that Chinese medicine teaches us the importance of strengthening and nourishing the kidneys so as to increase fertility? In both the male and female Essential Herbal Fertility Programs, I have included herbs that will do just that.

2. Unification of the mind and body of the couple during sex. If I see there is not true closeness between two partners, although they have agreed to have a child together, my hope is that they become closer as they begin the process of achieving pregnancy. How can a couple strengthen this "unification"? Practice looking into each other's eyes. Without speaking—no words, no gestures—set aside silent time to just stare into each other's "windows into the soul," in hopes of reaching and feeling what your partner feels, breaking down the "wall" between you. This may become very emotional for one or both parties. It may induce tears, even sobbing. If this occurs, I don't know of anyone who wouldn't reach out and comfort their partner with a loving, sensual embrace. This is needed. A couple must get back to the feelings they first felt for each other when they fell in love. This reemergence of closeness can help facilitate fertility.

3. Proper frequency of sex. Well, as I have already shared, having too much sex can harm sperm quality. During the time of strengthening and balancing both your bodies with the herbal therapy programs, lifestyle, and dietary changes, I recommend that the intimacy of sexual intercourse be reserved for the nine days during the woman's ovulation cycle to increase your chances of conception.

4. Avoidance of overwork, harshness, excessive sex and injury of genitals. Again, I will be blunt. The act of sex can be lively and enjoyed in infinite, inventive ways. For achieving conception, however, I feel that intercourse should be loving, slow and sensual with both of you looking into each other's eyes as much as possible. If there is overwork or harshness during sex, this will create stress, which we know is detrimental to one's balance and state of health. We are all adults here, so we should understand that rough sex is part of what many people enjoy. Again, however, this causes stress to the body, and not what I recommend when trying to conceive. The state of both your bodies, your physical, mental and emotional balance, are part of the makeup of your eggs and sperm. Do you want to pass on stressful chromosomes to your future baby? Pass on inner peace and love during your intimate sessions together. This will make for a more enriched baby-making experience.

5. Proper timing of orgasm. Something I feel is a marvelous benefit to creating a closer bond during sex is taking the time to let go slightly of the ego and just feel. Feeling your partner rising in pleasure during sexual intercourse, taking your time, moving in rhythm together, and waiting until both are about to achieve orgasm to explode in ecstasy in each other's arms. Although studies now show that a female orgasm is not necessary to conceive, female orgasm has been shown to help promote sperm transport. So take your time, rise and fall with each other, whisper in each other's ears what you are feeling during that wonderful time locked in pleasure with each other. Let each other know when you are both achieving your heights of pleasure, hold on, wait, and then explode in sexual rapture and climax together.

6. Expression of love and care during sex. I feel this continues to touch upon being gentle with each other before, during, and after intimacy. Foreplay that involves re-exploring each other's bodies, appreciating each other's skin, curves, muscles, delicateness, strength—all those physical attributes that attracted you both to each other in the first place—and again, looking into each other's eyes often, this enhances the love and care during sex.

7. Gentle and gradual intercourse. Yes, yes, yes! Remember, you are making a baby because you both truly care for and love each other. Shouldn't your lovemaking reflect that? I am sure you both also want your baby's makeup to be, every cell, of love.

8. Enhancement of energy in daily life to ensure male erectile function. Everything I've recommended will boost a man's energy (and a woman's energy, too). But, now that you know you should be intimate for 9 days straight to increase your chances of conception, does this sound stressful? We know now stress should be kept at bay because it affects our healthy physical balance and most definitely affects the health of the reproductive system.

However, to take advantage of strong male erection, a man should be stress-free, energized, and rested. For this reason, I advise couples to avoid trying to be intimate after a long, tiring, stressful day of work. The last thing you want is for sex to be viewed as a chore. For less stress and more energetic lovemaking during your 9-day 'baby-making marathon,' wake up early and have sex in the wee morning hours. For example, say you and your partner both normally wake up at 6:30 a.m. to get ready for your workday. Then, during your 9 days of baby-making, set a light sounding alarm, preferably with a musical tone you both find soothing for 5:00 a.m.

In your sleepiness, with already rested bodies, begin with affectionate touching and carry out this most dreamy time together with love emanating from both of your very souls. When finished, drift back to sleep in each other's arms until *your second alarm sounds at 6:30 a.m. Why is this so beneficial for male erectile function? Aside from stress being taken out of the equation, a healthy man, with healthy blood circulation, achieves his strongest erection in the morning. A man wakes up at 'attention' (like a soldier), and if he has a strong erection, sex is more pleasurable. When a man is rested enough to have a stress-free, strong erection during these 9 critical days, this improves the chances of conception.*

9. Health benefits through proper intercourse. *Of course, having sex is related to the, oh, so popular phrase, "if you don't use it, you lose it." Men are known to have between three to five erections per night, not including the erections that come about from sexual intimacy. Research from the Mayo College of Medicine supports that erections are vital to penile muscle health because they bring much-needed oxygen to the penis. Why is this so important?*

Sex is a healthy habit that helps to maintain nerve health. Furthermore, according to a study in the American Journal of Medicine, men who have sexual intercourse less than once a week are twice as likely to develop erectile dysfunction (ED). Yet, we must still keep in mind the factors of sperm quality. So, for the purpose of conception, outside of the 9-day 'marathon,' keep intercourse to one day a week to maintain good sexual health. And, what about for a woman? In a study published in the journal, Fertil Steril, sexual arousal was shown to increase blood flow and vaginal lubrication, which facilitates intercourse. And the more frequently a woman has sex the more she stimulates circulation to the genitals.

From my previous chapter on circulation, we know that good blood flow to the genital region is wonderful for increasing fertility and nourishing the reproductive system. This increase in blood flow then enhances lubrication and the elasticity of vaginal tissues. This goes hand-in-hand with boosting a woman's sexual pleasure and increasing fertility.

10. Sufficient rest after sex. Now see the reason why I recommend setting a gentle alarm to wake you both in the wee hours of the morning, when the body has sufficiently rested before sex, and after intimacy, allowing time to both hold each other for a while longer, resting once again, before beginning your daily routine and work day? Rest is necessary, in general, to have healthy, balanced bodies. In turn, this helps to increase fertility in both a man and a woman.

Now, I mention the morning time for lovemaking in response to the hectic and stressful world we live in. I've heard couples share with me, time and again, how one or both couples feel pressured and too exhausted to perform sexually after a hard day at work. So, the suggestion for morning intimacy works beautifully for these individuals. Then, we have those couples that prefer evening time alone to be sexual. Chinese medicine teaches that 'Circulation Sex' time is 7 p.m. to 9 p.m. This time interval belongs to the pericardium, the sack that protects the heart. The element that predominates here is fire energy.

The blood flow that runs in and out of the heart is regulated by the pericardium, and there is emotional energy related to it. Feelings of love, intimacy, affection, and sex, clearly show the emotional and physical connection with regards to the acts of sex. The blunt sexual, intimate energy of the kidneys and the love given off by the heart is moderated by the pericardium and this overall energy is most active during this specific two-hour time interval. If you are truly both rested, and feeling up to having loving sex during these evening hours then listen to your inner guidance and carry on with your desires! This will just bring additional flowing love circulating within you both during the process of making baby!

If these theories interest you, you can learn more from *The Yellow Emperor's Classic of Internal Medicine,* which covers traditional Chinese medicine practices that have become a landmark in the history of Chinese civilization. This text shares fundamental principles in the science of health preservation and an important view in the etiology of traditional Chinese medicine.

I hope all this brings a sense of relaxation when you think of the time you will both be intimate in making baby. It is meant to help you understand—from a naturopathic, truly Chinese, and yet natural point of view—how easy and joyful the process of overcoming fertility challenges and becoming parents can be.

Finally, let's touch upon the do's and dont's Chinese medicine emphasizes with respect to preserving health and sex. Anything that enhances our health preservation and increases sexual health will increase fertility in both a man and a woman.

Do not have sex during sundown, which, according to Chinese medicine, is the time when the kidney qi (chi) should be preserved. For this reason, again, I recommend you have intercourse during the 9-day ovulation cycle in the morning.

Do regularly eliminate as many toxins from the body as possible. As Chinese medicine teaches, it is best to urinate and evacuate the bowels before having sex.

Do enjoy sex with the body and the mind. This pertains to the bonding and connection formed through looking into each other's eyes, gentle touching, and slow foreplay. Do not have sex when one or both partners is sick. This is negative energy that can be transferred during sex and is not recommended, especially if trying to conceive.

Do not have sex when drunk, after having consumed even moderate alcohol, or under the influence of any stimulant or drug. This weakens the liver and kidney qi (chi) and, as I have shared with you, these organs must be balanced and healthy to increase fertility and maintain healthy reproductive systems.

Do not have sex on a full stomach or an empty stomach, both of which harm the qi (chi) and blood. Especially during the 9-day baby-making marathon, have a healthy dinner each night so your bodies are well nourished the next day when you are intimate in the early morning hours.

Do not have sex during a woman's menstruation. This, understandably, is a time when a woman is shedding 'toxic' blood, and nothing should interrupt this time by disturbing the menstrual flow of elimination.

There then is a risk of toxic blood being reabsorbed by the body and surrounding organs, causing fertility challenges and other reproductive system complications in the future. (The same reason why a woman should not use tampons.)

Do maintain clean genitals to avoid possibility of infection. This applies to both men and women. One beautiful way to maintain this Chinese medicine health preservation principle is to practice showering together often, every night if possible before bed, so you are both fresh for intimacy the next morning.

Do be intimate in quiet surroundings. If there is a television in your bedroom (which I strongly recommend you remove, as it is considered in Chinese medicine to be a negative energy in a place that should be for rest), then most definitely be sure not to fall asleep with the television on. Even if you have disruptive neighbors at night, then in the wee hours of the morning, when it is recommended you both take advantage of the 9-day ovulation cycle to make a baby, it should be peaceful enough for you to enjoy each other without distractions.

So, these are the last recommended steps to making baby. I hope The Naturopathic Approach to Fertility has given you fresh insights, but most importantly brought you the hope and comfort for which you and your partner have been so yearning. Now, take what you have learned here, take each other by the hand, feel the emotional desire you both have to make a beautiful miracle of your very own, and allow your bodies to be ready to receive. I am so very grateful to be a part of your journey and feel blessed to know this book has given you the tools to work with to make your dream of having a precious baby together a wonderful reality. Thank you.

~Dr. Julissa

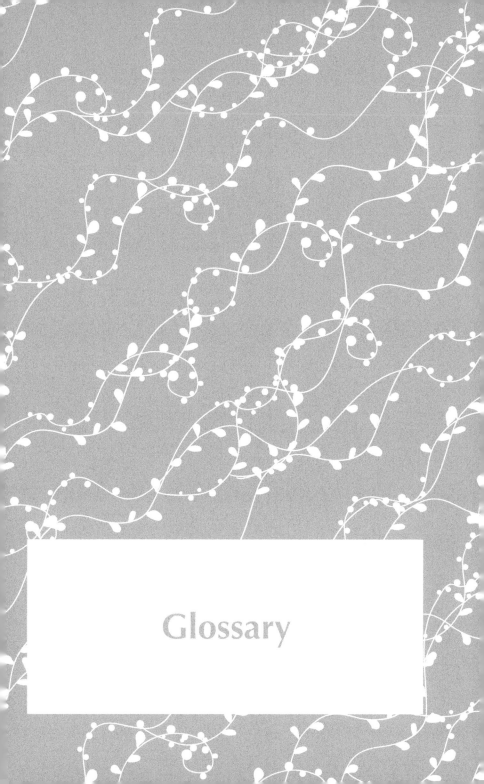

Glossary

Alfalfa

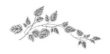

Parts used: Leaves

Forms available: Capsules (recommended), tablets, tinctures, teas

Use: Alfalfa is well known as the Father Herb because of its rich nutrient content. This herb is a common food plant for farm animals, but has a rich reputation in folk medicine for being a woman's herb—the mother's herb—promoting fertility, pregnancy, promoting the production of breast milk, increasing energy and boosting vitality. It is one of the herbs with the highest content of vitamins and minerals such as vitamins A, B6, B12, C, E, and K, as well as niacin and folate: a crucial nutrient known to help prevent birth defects in babies. It has also been used to relieve jaundice, encourage blood clotting, prevent heart disease, and help decrease the absorption of cholesterol. Alfalfa has been used throughout history for its immune-boosting qualities.

Recommended dosage: 340 mg per capsule (680 mg per 2 capsules). Take two capsules with a meal three times daily, or three capsules with a meal two times daily. Note: All recommended capsule dosages can be opened up in a glass of water as well.

Astragalus

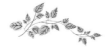

Parts used: Roots

Forms available: Capsules (recommended)

Use: Astragalus is a Chinese medicinal herb known as an adaptogenic tonic that strengthens the immune system and has been reputed to extend life span. It is a potent nutrient for the kidneys, which Chinese medicine teaches us is one of the secrets of longevity. This herb is also known in Chinese medicine to balance sugar levels in diabetics, lower blood pressure, act as an all-round stimulant for the immune system, strengthen those who feel weak, and boost health overall. Astragalus is an antiviral that is used to counteract immune-suppressing effects of cancer drugs and radiation, increase blood flow throughout the body, and reduces fluid retention. This herb also nourishes stressed, exhausted adrenal glands to fight lethargy and fatigue, increasing energy overall. It balances hormones while relaxing and normalizing the nervous system. This herb is commonly combined with other herbs in traditional Chinese medicine because it is believed to increase and promote the healing power of other remedies.

Recommended dosage: 420 mg per capsule (840 mg per 2 capsules). Take two capsules with a meal three times daily, or three capsules with a meal two times daily. Note: All recommended capsule dosages can be opened up in a glass of water as well.

Bayberry

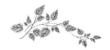

Parts used: Dried leaves, root

Forms available: Capsules (recommended), tea

Use: In the 1700s, this herb became popular as a remedy for fever, digestive problems, congestion, canker and oral health. Bayberry is an astringent on the intestinal membranes, drying up challenging diarrhea. It is warming and stimulates the circulatory system. Among fertility specialists, Bayberry is a well-known uterine tonic. It helps heal an inflamed uterus and is cherished for its potent affect on the lungs, bowels, and uterus by stopping hemorrhaging. It helps with clogged sinuses and is used by traditional naturopaths to help in fertility challenges involving blocked fallopian tubes. It is used to fortify the female reproductive system and balance liver health.

Recommended dosage: 440 mg per capsule. Take one capsule with a meal twice daily, or two capsules once a day.

Blessed Thistle

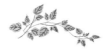

Parts used: Whole herb, aerial parts

Forms available: Capsules (recommended), tea

Use: Known as 'Mother's Herbal Helper,' this herb both wonderfully nourishes the reproductive system and is an excellent remedy for nursing mothers who seek to increase their breast milk production. Blessed Thistle enables a woman's breasts to produce more milk by promoting blood flow to the mammary glands, bringing in more nutrients and oxygen via the bloodstream. Use Blessed Thistle before conceiving to increase fertility. Once pregnancy is achieved, discontinue use. Resume Blessed Thistle intake after childbirth to support breastfeeding efforts. This herb is known for increasing liver function and fortifying the glandular system. This herb regulates a woman's menstrual period and promotes blood flow.

Recommended dosage: 325 mg per capsule (650 mg per 2 capsules). Take two capsules twice daily, or four capsules once a day.

Butcher's Broom

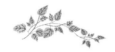

Parts used: Root

Forms available: Capsules (recommended)

Use: Butcher's Broom received its name in Europe when the prickly leaves were tied together to make brooms for cleaning butcher's blocks. This plant reduces hemorrhoids and inflammation while constricting the blood vessels of those with poor circulation, especially in the lower part of the body and the lower limbs. Overall, it is an excellent fortifier of the circulatory system.

Recommended dosage: 400 mg per capsule, (800 mg per 2 capsules). Take two capsules with a meal twice daily, or four capsules with a meal once a day.

Catnip

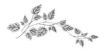

Parts used: Leaf

Forms available: Capsules (recommended), tincture, tea

Use: This herb is used as a relaxant. It is especially great for relaxing the body before bed and combats insomnia. Catnip strengthens the nervous system, helping one cope better with stress, and supports the immune system. It is rich in vitamins and minerals. Catnip has traditionally also been used to support the lungs and to help the body overcome respiratory ailments. For those who suffer from seizures and/or epilepsy, it has been used to prevent seizures, especially nighttime seizures.

Recommended dosage: 300 mg per capsule, (600 mg. per two capsules). Take two capsules with a meal three times daily, or three capsules with a meal two times daily.

Damiana

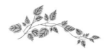

Parts used: Leaf

Forms available: Capsules (recommended), tea

Use: This herb has a reputation for being used by the Aztecs, men and women, as an aphrodisiac. It increases sexual desire while at the same time reducing tension, anxiety, and stress. Damiana increases blood flow to the pelvis, causing heightened arousal and enhancing sexual feelings and desire. It is a tonic of the reproductive system, especially the uterus, enhancing fertility. It has also been used as an antidepressant, to fight off fatigue, anxiety, exhaustion, and to increase energy. It supports sexual health, used by men to overcome impotence, premature ejaculation, and low libido (sexual desire). It increases sexual vitality and supports sexual performance in both males and females by strengthening the glandular system.

Recommended dosage: 350 mg per capsule, (700 mg per two capsules). Take two capsules with a meal twice daily, or four capsules once a day.

Dong Quai

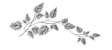

Parts used: Root

Forms available: Capsules (recommended), tinctures, tea

Use: Dong Quai increases blood flow to the uterus, thus increasing fertility. It helps ease painful menstruation, normalizes abnormal menstrual flow, promotes vitality, relieves fatigue, and strengthens the mother after childbirth. In Chinese medicine, it is often combined with Astragalus to strengthen and tone the kidneys. Dong Quai is also an herb that fortifies the immune system. It has been successfully used to reduce the deterioration of renal function and kidney damage. It has also been used as a nerve tonic, to relax the bowel, and to soothe the intestines. This herb also promotes blood flow to the reproductive system, and nourishes the blood.

Recommended dosage: 520 mg per capsule, (1040 mg per two capsules). Take two capsules with a meal three times daily, or three capsules with a meal twice daily.

Vitamin E with Selenium

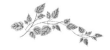

Parts used: Does not apply

Forms available: Softgel capsules (recommended), liquid

Use: This antioxidant is fat soluble, a vasodilator against blood clots and heart disease, and an anticoagulant. It protects cell membranes, destroys and neutralizes free radicals (which cause damage to cells), and improves brain function. Vitamin E works with selenium as an anti-aging supplement and lowers the risk of cancerous cell development. It promotes reproductive system health, increasing fertility in both men and women. It is a particularly excellent fertility aid for men, as vitamin E increases sperm motility and health. It also supports the circulatory system and helps normalize cholesterol levels. This supplement can also be used by women for vaginal dryness and as an excellent sexual lubricant. Pierce the softgel with a clean pin and squeeze the oil into the vagina daily and lubricate the men's penis to facilitate sex. Be sure to obtain natural vitamin E, also called d-alpha tocopherol, as opposed to synthetic vitamin E.

Recommended dosage: 400 IU (international units) of vitamin E, and 25 mcg of selenium, per capsule. To increase fertility, take one softgel capsule two times daily, or two softgel capsules once daily.

Gotu Kola

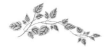

Parts used: Aerial parts

Forms available: Capsules (recommended), tincture, teas

Use: Gotu Kola is known to restore the nervous system, to treat neurotic problems, and is a potent relaxant. It is also known to increase libido (sexual desire). Gotu Kola has been used for increasing fertility, as it increases odds of conception. It has anti-aging effects and is considered within Chinese medicine as the 'fountain of youth.' It is known to improve focus, concentration and cognitive function. It also stabilizes mood by helping overcome anxiety. It is especially helpful for men to increase fertility by strengthening the seminiferous tubules by strengthening the connective tissue around blood vessels. This allows the sperm cell to mature and develop into viable spermatozoa ready to fertilize the egg. Gotu Kola is used to help balance hormones such as testosterone, maintains healthy sperm motility, encouraging sperm production and promoting sperm health overall.

Recommended dosage: 395 mg per capsule. Take one capsule with a meal three times daily, or three capsules once daily.

Grape Seed Extract

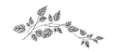

Parts used: Grape seed

Forms available: Capsules, tablets (both recommended)

Use: Grape Seed Extract is known to lower blood pressure and high cholesterol while treating other circulatory problems such as varicose veins and coronary heart disease. This potent anti-inflammatory supplement and powerful antioxidant has compounds that can help collect harmful byproducts of the body's many chemical processes existing within the brain. Grape Seed Extract helps alleviate asthma, allergies, and certain eye inflammation. It also helps balance blood sugar levels and prevents blood clots.

Recommended dosage: 25 mg per tablet. Take one tablet three times daily, or three tablets once daily.

Kelp

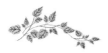

Parts used: Leaf and stem

Forms available: Capsules, tablets (both recommended), tincture, powder, liquid

Use: This well-known seaweed has been used in traditional Chinese medicine for thousands of years. It is rich in iodine, helping those with a sluggish thyroid gland manage weight gain. It is a natural thyroid stimulant and a rich source of essential trace minerals. It is a source of chlorophyll, and is effective in treating chronic sinus problems and gum disease. Kelp has been used to improve fertility in both men and women with great success. It increases energy, combats fatigue, enhances the functions of the liver, alleviates joint problems such as arthritis, prevents certain types of cancer and heart disease, suppresses AIDS and HIV, strengthens the immune system, and helps protect the body against the damaging effects of heavy metals and x-rays.

Recommended dosage: 525 mg per capsule (1050 mg per two capsules). Take two capsules with a meal twice daily, or four capsules once daily.

Lycopene

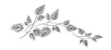

Parts used: Does not apply

Forms available: Capsules, tablets, softgels (all recommended)

Use: This is a well-known carotenoid because of its antioxidant properties. It protects against cancer, especially inhibiting prostate cancer. It is also known to strengthen immunity and protect the body against cancers of the digestive system, particularly the stomach and digestive tract. It has a history of showing very promising results in alleviating male infertility because it increases sperm count and viability. Lycopene reduces oxidative stress, therefore sperm is less vulnerable to oxidative damage, which increases the possibility of a normal sperm fertilizing an egg.

Recommended dosage: 4-8 mg per capsule. (Usually Lycopene is found in a proprietary blend combined with other herbs. My recommendation is a formula containing Standardaized Lycopene Concentrate in a proprietary blend of 1,224 mg per three capsules). Take three capsules twice daily.

Milk Thistle

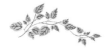

Parts used: Seed extract

Forms available: Capsules, tablets, (both recommended), tincture, softgels

Use: Another powerful antioxidant, Milk Thistle is revered for its healing powers in the treatment of liver-related disorders such as cirrhosis and hepatitis. It protects the precious liver from toxins including chemicals, drugs, and poisons. It neutralizes and detoxifies chemical pollutants and alcohol. The principle active ingredient, silymarin, helps in all the ailments mentioned here by reducing liver damage, helping in the treatment and prevention of gall bladder stones, and skin disorders such as psoriasis. A healthy liver is necessary for fertility. Using this herb increases the chances for conception in both men and women.

Recommended dosage: 175 mg per tablet, or 350 mg per two tablets. (This is also recommended in a formula combination containing this mg dosage.) Take two tablets with a meal twice daily.

Olive Leaf Extract

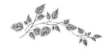

Parts used: Leaf

Forms available: Capsules, tablets (both recommended)

Use: Olive Leaf Extract is known as a powerful antiviral, anti-fungal, antibacterial, antiparasite, and antioxidant. It has been successfully used in helping the body fight off viruses in the treatment of herpes I and II, herpes virus 6 and 7, HIV and AIDS. It helps dispel chronic fatigue, the flu, colds, Epstein-Barr virus, shingles, meningitis, encephalitis, malaria, gonorrhea, pneumonia, tuberculosis, dental infection, chronic diarrhea, blood poisoning, urinary tract infections, ear infections, and infections that result from surgical procedures.

Recommended dosage: 420 mg per capsule. Take one capsule three times daily.

Pau D' Arco

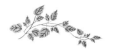

Parts used: Inner Bark

Forms available: Capsules (recommended), tincture, tea

Use: This Brazilian herb (Brazilian Taheebo Bark) is known as a natural hormone balancer used by the Inca and Maya civilizations. It has had success in helping those with certain cancers including leukemia. It gives the liver a healthy boost to function properly and balances women's hormones. It has been successful in helping those with muscle cramps, including severe menstrual cramps. Pau D'Arco is an herb often used to treat and help shrink abnormalities or accumulations of abnormal cells such as nodules, cysts, fibroids, etc. It is also used for all types of venereal diseases and candida albicans (yeast infections). Pau D'Arco has a supportive effect on the immune system as well.

Recommended dosage: 500 mg per capsule, or 1000 mg per 2 capsules. Take two capsules with a meal three times daily, or three capsules with a meal twice daily.

Queen Of The Meadow

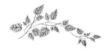

Parts used: Flowers, leaves, and entire plant

Forms available: Capsules (recommended), tinctures, tea

Use: This is a natural pain reliever and anti-inflammatory herb. It has been traditionally used for aches and pains of the joints, including those caused by gout, as well as for colds, bronchitis, the flu, headaches, and digestive complaints such as peptic ulcers, heartburn, and upset stomach. It also supports the urinary system by killing bacteria responsible for bladder infections. Traditionally, Queen of Meadow has been used to increase female fertility due to its function of helping to strengthen the female reproductive system overall.

Recommended dosage: This herb is most commonly found in formulations of a proprietary blend combined with other herbs. I recommend a proprietary blend including Queen of The Meadow at 400 mg per capsule, or 800 mg per two capsules. Take two capsules with a meal three times daily, or three capsules with a meal twice daily.

Red Raspberry Leaf

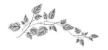

Parts used: Leaf

Forms available: Capsules (recommended), tablets, tinctures, teas

Use: The leaf of this favorite female remedy is one of the primary herbs in the Essential Female Herbal Therapy program. Often referred to as The Woman's Herb, it has been long used as a uterine toner and strengthener. It has been used in folk remedy for menstrual cramps, to regulate menstrual cycles, and to ease heavy menstrual periods. This herb should be used daily to nourish the female reproductive system, increasing fertility and preparing for conception and childbirth. A woman can continue use throughout her pregnancy to ease labor pains and relax uterine muscles before and during childbirth. Acting as an astringent, Red Raspberry Leaf has been known to help the body heal from wounds, diarrhea, mouth ulcers, gum inflammations, colds, and sore throats. It can also ease digestion and alleviate stomach ailments. It strengthens the kidneys as a cleansing diuretic, helping to ease also rheumatic problems. According to Chinese medicine, strengthening the kidneys strengthens the female reproductive system in turn.

Recommended dosage: 360 mg per capsule (720 mg per 2 capsules). Take two capsules with a meal three times daily, or three capsules with a meal twice daily.

St. John's Wort

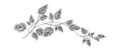

Parts used: Aerial parts

Forms available: Capsules, tablets (both recommended), tinctures, teas

Use: St. John's Wort is widely used to lift one's mood and spirit, initiating a feeling of enthusiasm. The liver benefits from this herb as it also helps cleanse and detoxify this vital organ. Anxiety, stress and depression are the main uses for this herb, and it provides incredible support to those suffering with these health challenges. St. John's Wort is known to be antiviral and so has been used successfully in the treatment of viral problems, most commonly the herpes virus, the flu virus (influenza), retroviruses (as in HIV), and Epstein-Barr. It strengthens, restores, and supports the nervous system and in this way minimizes the frequency of viral outbreaks during the healing process.

Recommended dosage: 300 mg. per capsule (900 mg per 3 capsules). Take one capsule with a meal three times daily, or three capsules with a meal once daily. Note: This herb is oftentimes wonderfully combined with other herbs such as Passion Flower, which enhances St. John's Wort's soothing effect as an anti-depressant, and is a support of the overall nervous system. Use before conception, not during pregnancy. Excessive exposure to sunlight or tanning beds during use is not recommended. Do not use combined with other pharmaceutical anti-depressant medications, amphetamines, blood thinners, bromocriptine, narcotic analgesics, pramipexole, or ropinirole. Do not use if you have taken a serotonin reuptake blocker within the last 14 days.

Saw Palmetto

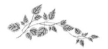

Parts used: Berries, leaf, stem

Forms available: Capsules, tablets (both recommended), tincture, tea

Use: Saw Palmetto has long been labeled a man's herb, although woman can use it as well. Tradition shows it has typically been used to treat infertility and as a male aphrodisiac. It strengthens and supports the prostate by alleviating an enlarged prostate, relieving prostate inflammation, correcting frequent nighttime urination, and strengthening the immune system. It is also very successful in treating urinary disorders.

Recommended dosage: 160 mg of saw palmetto berry extract concentrate per capsule. Take one capsule with a meal twice daily, or two capsules with a meal once daily.

Yarrow

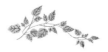

Parts used: Leaves, flowers

Forms available: Capsules (recommended), tincture, tea

Use: This herb is an astringent and helps the body recover from colds with its anti-catarrhal properties. It is a used with success as a diuretic, a stimulant of the digestive system, a peripheral vaso-dilator supporting the circulatory system, and a restorative of the female reproductive system by helping normalize menstruation. Yarrow is used as an anti-inflammatory for general healing and is found in many remedies to treat urinary challenges and colds.

Recommended dosage: 300 mg per capsule. Take one capsule with a meal twice daily, or two capsules once daily.

Zinc

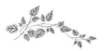

Parts used: Does not apply

Forms available: Capsule, tablets (both recommended), lozenge, liquid

Use: This is an essential mineral needed by everyone, by every cell in the human body. Zinc is found in concentrations in the pancreas, eyes, kidneys, liver, bones, muscles, and skin. It protects against free radical damage, is necessary for immune strength, and is known to be essential to the formation of insulin. It also supports the glands, reproductive and sexual health. By functioning on the immune system, zinc helps the body fight off flu, colds, conjunctivitis, and other types of infections. It helps prevent birth defects, increases the chances of healing, and improves eyesight by helping one overcome nearsightedness. Zinc also enhances sensory perception. It has even been known to aid in autoimmune disorders such as rheumatoid arthritis, fibromyalgia, lupus, and multiple sclerosis. Because of its potent effect on the immune system, it has shown promise in helping with such conditions as AIDS. One of zinc's most noted benefits is its effect on various hormones, including the sex and thyroid hormones. For this reason, zinc has always shown promise for enhancing fertility in both women and men. Zinc is recommended for those with glucose imbalances to help manage insulin levels, helping those with diabetes. Zinc may also support those with an under-active thyroid or an enlarged prostate.

Recommended dosage: Zinc can also be used in a formulation blend with other herbs and nutrients at 25 mg per tablet.

To increase fertility and double sperm count, it is recommended to consume at least 150 mg per day. Take two tablets with a meal three times daily, or three tablets with a meal twice daily.

To find all these supplements with the exact recommended levels and dosages I have recommended here, especially those in specific formulations, visit the Herbs & Supplements section of my website: www.DrJulissa.com.

Acknowledgements

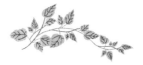

It is more than boundless gratitude that I have for all those involved with the radio show and television platforms I've been honored and humbled to be a part of over the years. You have inspired me, and were among the first ones to ever whisper in my ear, "You have to write a book…"

I wish to also thank my NSP Family for constantly drilling me with health questions, motivating me, and sharing numerous topics with me of books they wish for me to write.

And, lastly, I am infinitely grateful for being blessed with what I feel are the most supportive and loving team of experts in their field who helped me throughout the entire process of getting this final masterpiece in your hands (even during very late nights and holidays):

My amazing agent and publicist, Justin Loeber, Stephen Francy, and everyone at Mouth Public Relations for being here from the very beginning of the idea for this book; my sweet editor, Mysia Haight, for her warmth and understanding of my thoughts; and the marvelous, caring souls such as

Michelle Lewy, Marva Hinton, Hugo Villabona, Sofia Rodriguez, and everyone at Mango Publishing.

Thank you all for believing in me.

Thank you all for believing in this book. Thank you all for helping me share a part of me, a gift as this I can now share with the world, that I pray brings hope, happiness, health, and love for all time…

Author

Dr. Julissa Hernandez was introduced to natural medicine by her mother at a young age. Julissa grew up in poverty with her parents and two sisters in a small three-room apartment in the Bronx. There wasn't much money for prescription medicine, and the family depended on alternative methods, such as simple teas made from herbs and roots to help the body heal. That cursory knowledge ignited a fiery curiosity to look up an array of herbs and roots in the encyclopedia and to learn their healing properties. She read voraciously, and while still in high school, she attended natural health courses alongside her mother. This excitement eventually led her to seek certification and degrees beginning with general studies at New York University, then her registered certification as a CNHP (Certified Natural Health Professional) from the National Association of Certified Natural Health Professionals, Inc., and her ND (Doctorate Degree in Naturopathy), making her a nationally registered Doctor of Naturopathy from Trinity College of Natural Health in Warsaw, Indiana.

She's been practicing natural medicine for the past 21 years. A master in her field as a classical herbalist and holistic iridologist, she founded The Natural Health Center Inc. in New York City as her home office to see patients and clients. Now, she travels throughout the U.S. and abroad to consult personally with patients.

Dr. Julissa has served as a keynote speaker at health conferences and conventions, both domestically and internationally, and she has been a frequent guest on radio and television. For nine years, she was the resident official Naturopathic Doctor of the nationally syndicated radio program, 'The Michael Baisden Show' on the weekly segment 'Your Body Is Your Temple.' She's also a frequent special guest of national and international television, radio and online media including Telemundo and Blog Talk Radio. Since 2013, she's been featured live weekly as the official resident Naturopathic Doctor of two radio shows: 'To Your Good Health Thursdays' on WGLRO.com Radio and 'Healthy Living with Dr. Julissa' on Source Radio Network.

She's been called the modern day herbal authority on male and female reproductive system health, emotional wellbeing, anti-aging and beauty.

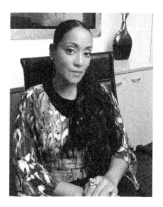

CPSIA information can be obtained at www.ICGtesting.com
Printed in the USA
BVOW05s0303180816

459387BV00003B/4/P